Drug Epidemiology and
Post-Marketing Surveillance

NATO ASI Series

Advanced Science Institutes Series

A series presenting the results of activities sponsored by the NATO Science Committee, which aims at the dissemination of advanced scientific and technological knowledge, with a view to strengthening links between scientific communities.

The series is published by an international board of publishers in conjunction with the NATO Scientific Affairs Division

A	**Life Sciences**	Plenum Publishing Corporation
B	**Physics**	New York and London
C	**Mathematical and Physical Sciences**	Kluwer Academic Publishers
D	**Behavioral and Social Sciences**	Dordrecht, Boston, and London
E	**Applied Sciences**	
F	**Computer and Systems Sciences**	Springer-Verlag
G	**Ecological Sciences**	Berlin, Heidelberg, New York, London,
H	**Cell Biology**	Paris, Tokyo, Hong Kong, and Barcelona
I	**Global Environmental Change**	

Recent Volumes in this Series

Volume 218—Pharmaceutical Applications of Cell and Tissue Culture to Drug Transport
edited by Glynn Wilson, S. S. Davis, L. Illum, and Alain Zweibaum

Volume 219—Atherosclerotic Plaques: Advances in Imaging for Sequential Quantitative Evaluation
edited by Robert W. Wissler

Volume 220—The Superfamily of *ras*-Related Genes
edited by Demetrios A. Spandidos

Volume 221—New Trends in Pharmacokinetics
edited by Aldo Rescigno and Ajit K. Thakur

Volume 222—The Changing Visual System: Maturation and Aging in the Central Nervous System
edited by P. Bagnoli and W. Hodos

Volume 223—Mechanisms in Fibre Carcinogenesis
edited by Robert C. Brown, John A. Hoskins, and Neil F. Johnson

Volume 224—Drug Epidemiology and Post-Marketing Surveillance
edited by Brian L. Strom and Giampaolo Velo

Series A: Life Sciences

Drug Epidemiology and Post-Marketing Surveillance

Edited by

Brian L. Strom

University of Pennsylvania
Philadelphia, Pennsylvania

and

Giampaolo Velo

University of Verona
Verona, Italy

Plenum Press
New York and London
Published in cooperation with NATO Scientific Affairs Division

Proceedings of a NATO Advanced Study Institute
on Drug Epidemiology and Post-Marketing Surveillance,
held September 27–October 8, 1990,
in Erice, Sicily, Italy

Library of Congress Cataloging-in-Publication Data

NATO Advanced Study Institute on Drug Epidemiology and Post-Marketing
    Surveillance (1990 : Erice, Italy)
    Drug epidemiology and post-marketing surveillance / edited by
Brian L. Strom and Giampaolo Velo.
        p.   cm. -- (NATO ASI series. Series A, Life sciences ; v.
    224)
    "Proceedings of a NATO Advanced Study Institute on Drug
Epidemiology and Post-Marketing Surveillance, held September
27-October 8, 1990, in Erice, Sicily, Italy"--T.p. verso.
    "Published in cooperation with NATO Scientific Affairs Division."
    Includes bibliographical references and index.
    ISBN 0-306-44099-7
    1. Pharmacoepidemiology--Congresses. 2. Drugs--Marketing-
-Congresses.   I. Strom, Brian L.   II. Velo, G. P. (Giampaolo)
III. North Atlantic Treaty Organization. Scientific Affairs
Division. IV. Title. V. Series.
    [DNLM: 1. Drug Evaluation--congresses. 2. Epidemiologic Methods-
-congresses. 3. Product Surveillance, Postmarketing--methods-
-congresses.   QV 771 N2792d 1990]
RM302.5.N38   1990
363.19'4--dc20
DNLM/DLC
for Library of Congress   91-45569
                                                                 CIP

ISBN 0-306-44099-7

© 1992 Plenum Press, New York
A Division of Plenum Publishing Corporation
233 Spring Street, New York, N.Y. 10013

Printed in the United States of America

PREFACE

This volume is a summary of material presented in the course given in the International School of Pharmacology on "Drug Epidemiology and Post-Marketing Surveillance" between September 27 and October 8, 1990, at the "Ettore Majorana Center for Scientific Culture" in Erice, Sicily. The course, which was a NATO Advanced Study Institute, included lectures and workshops presented by experts in the new field of pharmacoepidemiology. The material covered includes various approaches to spontaneous reporting of adverse drug reactions, including aggregate approaches, such as those used in France, and detailed analyses of individual reports, such as that done in The Netherlands and in Sweden. Also, included are studies using traditional epidemiology methods. In addition, modern pharmacoepidemiology makes considerable use of automated databases. As such, information is presented on their use as well. Pharmacoepidemiology started in hospitals and some of the newest work in the field is returning to the hospital as a site for studies. Material on these topics was presented as well. Finally, selected new methodologic developments were outlined in specific examples presented that were of regulatory and commercial importance.

This new field of pharmacoepidemiology is exploding in interest internationally. Evidence of this is the increasing development of pharmacoepidemiology programs in industry, medical schools, pharmacy schools, and schools of public health. Also, there is a new International Society of Pharmacoepidemiology.

Practitioners in this field tend to specialize in either analyses of spontaneous reporting or the use of formal epidemiologic techniques. Part of the goal of this course was to cross-fertilize these two branches of pharmacoepidemiology. It is hoped that this book will be useful in encouraging the continued development of this field and the continued cross-fertilization of these branches.

Finally, we would like to take this opportunity to express our gratitude to all the invited speakers for their contributions to the course and also for their ability to create an atmosphere conducive to informal learning.

Brian L. Strom, M.D., M.P.H.
Giampaolo Velo, M.D.

CONTENTS

SECTION A
SPONTANEOUS REPORTING

The Analysis of Postmarketing Drug Surveillance Data
      at the U.S. Food and Drug Administration 1
   Thomas P. Gross, M.D., M.P.H.

Postmarketing Surveillance of ADRs by Spontaneous Reporting
      and Register Data: The Swedish Approach 9
   Bengt-Erik Wiholm, M.D., Ph.D.

Spontaneous Monitoring of Adverse Reactions to Drugs,
      Procedures, and Experiences in The Netherlands 21
   R.H.B. Meyboom, M.D.

Pharmacovigilance in France: A Decentralized Approach 39
   Bernard Begaud, M.D.

SECTION B
TRADITIONAL CLINICAL EPIDEMIOLOGY METHODS
AS APPLIED TO PHARMACOEPIDEMIOLOGY

The Use of Vital and Morbidity Statistics for the Detection
      of Adverse Drug Reactions and for Monitoring of Drug Safety 43
   Paul D. Stolley, M.D., M.P.H.

The Use of Case-Control Studies in Pharmacoepidemiology 49
   Paul D. Stolley, M.D., M.P.H.

The Use of Cohort Studies in Pharmacoepidemiology 53
   Terri H. Creagh, M.S., M.S.P.H.

Using Randomized Trials in Pharmacoepidemiology 59
   Gordon H. Guyatt, M.D.

SECTION C
USE OF AUTOMATED DATABASES FOR PHARMACOEPIDEMIOLOGY

Pharmacoepidemiology Studies Using Large Databases 65
   Brian L. Strom, M.D., M.P.H.

Screening for Unknown Effects of Newly Marketed Drugs 73
    Jeffrey L. Carson, M.D. and Brian L. Strom, M.D., M.P.H.

SECTION D
HOSPITAL PHARMACOEPIDEMIOLOGY

Hospital Data Sources 83
    Judith K. Jones, M.D., Ph.D.

Hospital-Based Intensive Cohort Studies 91
    Keith Beard, B.Sc., M.B.

Hospital-Based Adverse Reaction and Drug Utilization Review
    in the United States 99
    Brian L. Strom, M.D., M.P.H.

SECTION E
NEW METHODOLOGIC DEVELOPMENTS

Approaches to Evaluating Causation of Suspected Drug Reactions 103
    Judith K. Jones, M.D., Ph.D.

Pharmacoeconomics: Principles and Basic Techniques
    of Economic Analysis 115
    Henry Glick, M.A. and Raynard Kington, M.D.

N of 1 Randomized Trials for Investigating New Drugs 125
    Gordon H. Guyatt, M.D.

Measuring Health-Related Quality of Life in Clinical Trials 135
    Gordon H. Guyatt, M.D.

SECTION F
SELECTED EXAMPLES OF REGULATORY AND COMMERCIAL IMPORTANCE

Evaluation of Bias and Validation of Survival Estimates
    in a Large Cohort of AIDS Patients Treated with Zidovudine 143
    Terri H. Creagh, M.S., M.S.P.H.

The Triazolam Experience in 1979 in The Netherlands,
    a Problem of Signal Generation and Verification 159
    R.H.B. Meyboom, M.D.

Contributors 169

Index 171

THE ANALYSIS OF POSTMARKETING DRUG SURVEILLANCE DATA

AT THE U.S. FOOD AND DRUG ADMINISTRATION

Thomas P. Gross, M.D., M.P.H.

Office of Epidemiology and Biostatistics
Food and Drug Administration
Rockville, Maryland 20857

Surveillance of adverse drug reactions (ADRs) may be defined as the systematic ascertainment of drug-induced illness by practical uniform methods.[1] Various strategies have been proposed for postmarketing surveillance of these illnesses.[2,3] For example, Jick categorized these strategies on the bases of the underlying illness rates and the rates of adverse reactions attributable to drugs.[3] He suggested that spontaneous ADR reporting systems would be most effective in their surveillance when the actual ADR rate is high and the underlying rate of the illness in the population is low. Thalidomide-induced phocomelia is a good example of this type of drug-related adverse reaction. If the ADR rate is low and the background rate of the illness in the general population is high, observational studies like case-control or cohort studies rather than spontaneous reporting would be needed to identify and characterize the risk of drug-induced illness.

The U.S. Food and Drug Administration (FDA) has conducted postmarketing surveillance and analysis of drug-related adverse reactions for many years. This paper presents some of the methods used in the aggregate analyses of spontaneously reported ADRs at the FDA and related statistical issues, preceded by a brief description of the surveillance system and its limitations.

THE EXISTING DATABASE

Since the mid-1960s, the FDA has received, evaluated, and processed over 450,000 reports of ADRs. Of the 50,000-60,000 reports received annually, approximately 90% originate from manufacturers and the remaining 10% from health care providers and consumers.[4] These reports are submitted on a standardized FDA Form-1639. The information collected includes patient initials or identification number, age, sex, date of birth, reaction onset date, description of the reaction, relevant laboratory values, suspect and concomitant drugs, and information about the suspect drug, including manufacturer, indication for its use, and dates of administration.

Each report is entered into the FDA's computerized spontaneous reporting system database using a coding thesaurus of ADR terms to code the reaction for retrieval purposes.[5] The coding terminology aids in the grouping of reports by ADR term(s) or by organ systems. About 15 working days elapse between receipt of reports of most concern (i.e., serious unlabelled reports either from manufacturers or directly from health professionals) and their computerization. Serious reactions are defined as those that are life-threatening; result in either death, permanent disability, or inpatient hospitalization; or are congenital anomalies or malignancies. Further details on the database are provided elsewhere.[4]

Drug Epidemiology and Post-Marketing Surveillance, Edited by B.L. Strom
and G. Velo, Plenum Press, New York, 1992

LIMITATIONS OF THE DATABASE

The existing database has limitations which should be taken into account in any interpretation of aggregate analyses of ADR reports. The most obvious limitations are underreporting, reporting biases, uncertain causality, inadequate information, and inability to accurately quantitate drug use (i.e., to estimate the population at risk).

Underreporting results from an inability to detect a reaction, to attribute a reaction to a drug, or to report a reaction to the FDA (or the manufacturer). Even unusual and serious possible ADRs have historically been highly underreported.[6,7]

Reporting biases have been associated with the year in the marketing life of a drug (i.e., rates vary with the newness of the drug)[8], secular trends in reporting (i.e., generally increased reporting of ADRs for more recently marketed drugs)[9], manufacturer reporting practices (including size and training of manufacturer's sales force)[10], publicity (including advertising, special promotions, Dear Doctor letters, articles in the medical literature and lay press)[11], pending litigation, and the uniqueness or severity of the reaction.

Causal uncertainty may result from confounding by indication (i.e., the illness being treated or concomitant illnesses may themselves cause the suspected reaction), from confounding due to the presence of concomitant drugs or other exposures (e.g., alcohol, smoking) known to be associated with the reaction, from lack of certain information (e.g., information on rechallenge to the suspect drug), and from difficulties in establishing temporal relationships between exposure and reaction (especially true for reactions that have relatively long latent periods).

Finally, there is difficulty in identifying the population at risk. Often, the only estimates of the population risk will be based on estimates of drug use, currently provided to the FDA by IMS America.[12] These estimates of the population at risk are used in conjunction with ADR reports to compute reporting rates. It is important to keep in mind that reporting rates are not incidence rates for reasons noted above.

Despite these limitations, the FDA's ADR database has utility as an early warning system to signal a previously unknown ADR, especially when the reaction is relatively unusual, frequent, and occurs in close temporal relationship to exposure. It has been noted that most unexpected ADRs are discovered by voluntary reporting.[13]

ADR monitoring can serve as a means of profiling the types of adverse reactions likely to be found with a given drug and provide information about host susceptibility factors. For example, nonsteroidal antiinflammatory ADR reports indicate that butazones are more likely to be associated with hematologic adverse reactions than other drugs in the class and that elderly women are at greatest risk.[14] Finally, ADR surveillance can be used in the aggregate analyses of ADRs to identify an increase in frequency of previously known or unknown drug-related reactions.

The use of FDA adverse reaction reports in relation to the discovery of new ADRs has been previously investigated. Compared to three postmarketing observational cohort studies which detected no new ADRs (for the drugs cimetidine, cyclobenzaprine, and prazosin), the FDA's ADR database was able to identify new ADRs for two of the three study drugs.[15] In another study, the effectiveness of the database in identifying new ADRs (expressed as the percentage of new ADRs that subsequently became part of the labelling) was examined.[16] The authors concluded that the FDA's ADR reporting system, particularly reports received directly from physicians, was capable of making a contribution to the identification of new ADRs.

AGGREGATE ANALYSES

Recent improvements in the processing of FDA ADR reports has increased the opportunity for aggregate analyses of drug-related reactions. Currently, the two basic approaches being used at the FDA are: (a) comparing the frequency of reports for a drug relative to itself in previous time periods, and (b) comparing the frequency of reports for a drug with other drugs in the same therapeutic class (adjusted for various reporting factors). These analyses should generally be considered as crude estimates and seen as signals, even when appropriate adjustments for potential biases are made. As our understanding of the limitations of the ADR database improves, more sophisticated techniques will hopefully be developed and utilized as well.

Comparing Reports for a Drug Relative to Itself in Previous Time Periods

The 1985 modification to the New Drug Regulations[17] requires the manufacturer of an approved new drug to submit to the FDA all drug reports quarterly for the first three years of marketing and annually thereafter, and to evaluate whether or not an increased frequency of serious known (labelled) reactions has occurred over comparable time periods. The regulations recognize that an increased frequency of adverse reaction reports may be related to an increasing number of patients exposed to the drug, so that an increased frequency is not to be assessed unless adjustments for exposure estimates can be made.

Suppose a recently approved drug is known from clinical experience in premarketing studies to produce agranulocytosis. During the third quarter, 81 reports of agranulocytosis were received, while 20 reports were received during the previous second quarter. Suppose that an estimated 40,000 prescriptions were written during the third quarter as compared with 30,000 prescriptions during the second quarter. The fundamental assumption of this first method of analysis is that the number of reports received during the third quarter should be proportional to the number of reports received during the second quarter, when account is taken of the estimated drug use during these two quarters. Thus, the expected number of reports in the third quarter, if such proportionality holds, would be $20 \times (40,000/30,000) = 27$.

The FDA has asked to be notified by manufacturers when they observe more than a doubling of the expected number of reports during a reporting period (whether it be quarterly, semi-annually, annually), after account is taken of changes in drug use. In this example, that should have occurred if 54 or more reports were received in the third quarter.

The FDA recognizes that the doubling criteria is arbitrary. Alternate statistically based procedures which better account for the variability in reporting from period to period and which can better assess time trends among reporting periods can also be used.

Comparing Reports for Drugs in the Same Therapeutic Class Adjusting for Various Reporting Factors

Because of the FDA's unique position as a repository for all ADR reports in the U.S., the FDA has available to it adverse reaction reports submitted by all manufacturers who have drugs in a similar therapeutic drug class. Methods have been developed which utilize estimates of drug usage to identify those drugs which may have reports in excess of that which might be expected given the relative drug use or market share.

The use of the ADR database for this comparative purpose has some of the inherent difficulties previously mentioned with regard to reporting biases. These difficulties include reporting that varies with the year in the marketing life of a drug, secular trends in reporting, manufacturer reporting practices, publicity, pending litigation, and changing FDA procedures for processing incoming reports. Any comparison of drugs in a therapeutic class must take these factors into account.

The following example illustrates the use of ADR reports for two drugs in a therapeutic class in conjunction with their estimates of drug use during similar years in their marketing life (Table 1A). Assume that A1 and A2 are the number of reports of adverse reactions associated with Drugs 1 and 2, respectively. Then assume that Drug 1 has N1 as the estimate of drug use (e.g., numbers of prescriptions) and that Drug 2 has N2 as its estimate. The estimates of the proportion of usage can be calculated as $Q1=N1/N3$ and $Q2=N2/N3$ for each drug respectively, where $N3=N1+N2$. The standardized reporting ratio (SRR) for each drug is defined as the ratio of the observed number of reports to the expected number of reports for that drug. The latter is the product of the total number of reports (A3) and its proportional drug use in the therapeutic class. Thus, the SRR for Drug 1 is $A1/(A3 \times Q1)$ and the SRR for Drug 2 is $A2/(A3 \times Q2)$, where $A3=A1+A2$.

The magnitude of the SRR for each drug is used by FDA as an indicator to possibly investigate each drug further, particularly those drugs whose SRR's are substantially higher (or lower) than one, meaning that the number of reports received for that drug deviates from what might be expected given its market share within its therapeutic class.

The statistical sampling variation of the SRR can be calculated and used to construct statistical confidence intervals which account for the variability in number of reports and help in assessing the range of SRR's consistent with the observed data.

The SRR can also be derived in an analogous manner with a method utilizing reporting rates (Table 1B). By this method, the expected number of reports for a drug is the product of the overall reporting rate (RR3) and its estimate of drug use.

Table 1.   The Standardized Reporting (SRR*) Ratio for Comparison Drugs during Similar Years in Their Marketing Life

	Drug 1	Drug 2	Total
Years in marketing life (1st through 3rd)	1980-1982	1985-1987	

A.   *Total number of reports and percentage of drug use*

	Drug 1	Drug 2	Total
Reports	A1 10	A2 4	A3=A1+A2 14
Drug use	N1 40,000	N2 60,000	N3=N1+N2 100,000
Percentage of use	Q1 0.40	Q2 0.60	Q3=Q1+Q2 1.00
Expected reports	A1^=A3xQ1 5.6=14x0.40	A2^=A3xQ2 8.4=14x0.60	
(SRR*)	SRR1=A1/A1^ 1.79=10/5.6	SRR2=A2/A2^ 0.48=4/8.4	

B.   *Overall reporting rate and drug use*

	Drug 1	Drug 2	Total
Reporting rate	RR1=A1/N1 2.5×10^{-4}	RR2=A2/N2 6.7×10^{-5}	RR3=A3/N3 1.4×10^{-4}
Expected reports	A1^=RR3xN1 5.6	A2^=RR3xN2 8.4	
(SRR*)	SRR1=A1/A1^ 1.79=10/5.6	SRR2=A2/A2^ 0.48=4/8.4	

*SRR: observed number of reports/expected number of reports

Reporting rates for a specific drug in comparison with other drugs in the same class can be further refined with attention given to initial year of marketing of each drug (to adjust for secular trends in reporting) and to other factors that may contribute to reporting bias (e.g., differences in manufacturer reporting).   For example, using the hypothetical adjustments for secular trend and manufacturer reporting noted in Table 2, the adjusted reporting rate ratio (RR1**/RR2**) would be 2.22 compared to the unadjusted value (RR1/RR2) of 3.73. As with the SRR, the reporting rate ratio can also provide a crude signal for further investigation; again, particularly for ratios whose values substantially deviate from one.

Table 2.   The Reporting Rate and Rate Ratio Adjusted for Secular Trend and
            Manufacturer Reporting

	Drug 1	Drug 2
Years in marketing life (1st through 3rd)	1980-1982	1985-1987
Year of initial marketing	1980	1985
Manufacturer	Y	Z
Reporting rate^	$RR1=A1/N1$ 2.5×10^{-4}	$RR2=A2/N2$ 6.7×10^{-5}
Reporting rate ratio	$RRR1=RR1/RR2$ 3.73	$RRR2=RR2/RR1$ 0.27
Secular trend adjustment#	$RR1^*=RR1 \times 1$ 2.5×10^{-4}	$RR2^*=RR2/1.5$ 4.5×10^{-5}
Manufacturer reporting adjustment~	$R1^{**}=RR1^*/2.5$ 1×10^{-4}	$RR2^{**}=RR2^* \times 1$ 4.5×10^{-5}
Adjusted reporting rate ratio	$RRR1^*=RR1^{**}/RR2^{**}$ 2.22	$RRR2^*=RR2^{**}/RR1^{**}$ 0.45

^See tables 1A and 1B.
#Assumes that 1980 is the referent year and that the 1985 all drug-reporting rate is 1.5 times as great as the 1980 rate.
~Assumes that manufacturer Z is the referent manufacturer and that Y's reporting rate for this therapeutic class of drugs is 2.5 times as great as Z's.

STATISTICAL ISSUES

Finney[18] has written on the use of spontaneous reporting as a method for monitoring ADRs. Finney stressed five key assumptions on which aggregate analyses will be based, namely independence, representativeness, susceptibility equivalence, background equivalence, and unbiased reporting. Consideration of these assumptions should help place proposed analyses in a proper perspective.

Independence exists when the report of one adverse reaction does not influence the report of another adverse reaction, for the drug of interest or any comparison drug. Independence implies that reports of ADRs for a drug does not influence the additional reporting of ADRs for that drug.

Representativeness exists when exposures to drugs within a given drug class noted in ADR reports of interest are similar in proportion to exposures in the population with the ADR. Susceptibility equivalence exists when the inherent possibility of a specific adverse reaction occurring (independent of any drug effect) is the same for two or more drugs in the same class.

Background equivalence implies that the observed difference is not due to unique patient characteristics or the result of patient care. Unbiased reporting implies that the reaction being reported does not depend upon the drug, as might be the case if a drug has had recent adverse publicity.

In any application of aggregate analyses, one needs to consider whether or not the available data comply at least approximately to these underlying assumptions.

CONCLUSION

This paper has pointed out some of the methods that can be used for aggregate analyses of ADRs and has discussed how the validity of any analysis will depend on the validity of the underlying assumptions, the reliability of drug use data, and the quality of the reports. The FDA believes that the spontaneous ADR reporting system, with emphasis on analyses of aggregate reports, continues to be a valuable tool for the surveillance of marketed drugs. Surveillance does not guarantee that drugs will be safe but it does provide a means by which adverse reactions to drugs can be identified and appropriate measures taken.

ACKNOWLEDGEMENT

This manuscript is based on a presentation made at the American Public Health Association Meeting in Washington, D.C. in November 1985. The presentation, authored by Charles Anello, Sc.D. and Robert O'Neill, Ph.D. of the Office of Epidemiology and Biostatistics of the Food and Drug Administration, was entitled "The analysis of postmarketing drug surveillance data."

DISCLAIMER

This paper contains the professional views of the author and does not constitute the official position of the Food and Drug Administration.

REFERENCES

1.   G. A. Faich, Adverse-drug-reaction monitoring, *N Eng J Med*. 314:1589-92 (1986).
2.   D. J. Finney, Systematic signalling of adverse reactions to drugs, *Meth Inf Med*. 13:1-10 (1974).
3.   H. Jick, The discovery of drug-induced illness, *N Eng J Med*. 290:481-5 (1977).
4.   J. M. Sills, A. Tanner, and J. B. Milstien, Food and Drug Administration monitoring of adverse drug reactions, *Am J Hosp Pharm*. 43:2764-70 (1986).
5.   W. T. Turner, J. B. Milstien, G. A. Faich, and G. D. Armstrong, The processing of adverse reaction reports at FDA, *Drug Inf J*. 20:147-50 (1986).
6.   P. Arneborn, J. Palmblad, Drug-induced neutropenia--a survey for Stockholm: 1973-1978, *Acta Med Scand*. 212:289-92 (1982).
7.   W. H. W. Inman, Study of fatal bone marrow depression with special reference to phenylbutazone and oxyphenylbutazone, *Brit Med J*. 1:1500-5 (1977).
8.   J. C. P. Weber, Epidemiology of adverse reactions to nonsteroidal antiinflammatory drugs, *in*: "Advances in inflammation research," K. D. Rainsford, and G. P. Velo, eds., Vol 6., Raven Press, New York (1984).
9.   A. C. Rossi, J. P. Hsu, and G. A. Faich, Ulcerogenicity of piroxicam: an analysis of spontaneously reported data, *Br Med J*. 294:147-50 (1987).
10.   C. Baum, G. A. Faich GA, Anello C, Forbes MB, Differences in manufacturer reporting of adverse drug reactions to the FDA in 1984, *Drug Inf J*. 21:257-66 (1987).
11.   A. C. Rossi, L. Bosco, G. A. Faich, A. Tanner, and R. Temple, The importance of adverse reaction reporting by physicians: Suprofen and flank pain syndrome, *JAMA*. 259;1203-4 (1988).
12.   IMS America, Ltd. Plymouth Meeting, Pa.
13.   Medicine in the public interest: postmarketing surveillance of drugs, Report of the Conference, Washington, D.C., October 29-31 (1976).

14. J. K. Jones, Regulatory use of adverse drug reactions, *in*: "Skandia International Symposia: detection and prevention of adverse drug reactions," Almquist International, Stockholm, 203-14 (1984).

15. A. C. Rossi, D. E. Knapp, C. Anello C, and et al., Discovery of new adverse drug reactions, a comparison of phase IV studies with spontaneous reporting methods, *JAMA*. 249:2226-8 (1983).

16. A. C. Rossi, and D. E. Knapp, Discovery of new adverse drug reactions, a review of the Food and Drug Administration's spontaneous reporting system, *JAMA*. 252:1030-3 (1984).

17. Federal Register, New Drug and Antibiotic Regulations: Final Rule (February 22, 1985).

18. D. J. Finney, Statistical logic in the monitoring of reactions to therapeutic drugs, *Meth Inf Med*. 10:237-45 (1971).

POSTMARKETING SURVEILLANCE OF ADRs BY SPONTANEOUS REPORTING AND REGISTER DATA: THE SWEDISH APPROACH

Bengt-Erik Wiholm, M.D., Ph.D.

Section of Pharmacoepidemiology
Medical Products Agency
Uppsala, Sweden

Before a new drug is allowed on the market it has been thoroughly tested, first in animals and later in healthy volunteers and in patients. Thus, most of its positive effects and the more common adverse effects are known. However, because of the inherent limitations in premarketing testing with regard to population size and composition, and the limited number of long-term studies available, the full profile of positive and negative effects of a new drug cannot be known prior to marketing. It is therefore of utmost importance that new drugs be continuously monitored for new effects. The objective of postmarketing surveillance (PMS) is therefore to make inferences about new drug-related effects; traditionally PMS studies focus on adverse effects.

The process of evaluating new adverse effects is outlined in Table 1. Each of these steps calls for a method which is fine tuned to the specific problem. This means that we must have a wide array of methods at hand and that no single method can answer all relevant questions. Examples of such methods are pharmaco-kinetic, -dynamic and -genetic studies, randomized clinical trials, cohort studies, and case-control studies. Moreover, we need several data sources to which the methods can be applied, e.g., spontaneous reporting, case records, interviews, enquiries, and registries.

Spontaneous reports have hitherto been the most effective data source for the detection of new suspected adverse drug reactions (ADRs).[1-3] The hypotheses raised can sometimes be verified or refuted by experimental methods using single or small series of patients, but most often -- especially for idiosyncratic reactions -- this must be done on a population level by establishing a significant increase in relative and excess risks.

In this chapter I will describe some of the methods and data sources available in Sweden (Table 2) and give some examples of how they can be used. I will focus on the cohort method and the use of spontaneous reports and registers as data sources. I will emphasize the importance of close case analysis for valid results.

THE SPONTANEOUS REPORTING SYSTEM

Voluntary reporting by physicians and dentists of suspected adverse drug reactions started in Sweden in 1965, and since 1975 the reporting of fatal, otherwise serious, and new reactions has been compulsory. The reports are scrutinized for completeness by a medical officer who is a pharmacist or a physician and the full medical records, including laboratory tests and autopsies, are requested for all fatal cases and for the majority of those otherwise serious. The reports are then discussed and evaluated by a working party and, finally, by the Swedish Adverse Drug Reactions Advisory Committee, which has representatives from seven clinical specialties.

Drug Epidemiology and Post-Marketing Surveillance, Edited by B.L. Strom and G. Velo, Plenum Press, New York, 1992

Table 1. The Process of Evaluating New Adverse Drug Reactions (ADRs)

* Detection of a potential adverse effect and the formulation of an hypothesis
* Verification or refutation of the hypothesis
* Exploration of mechanisms in search of potential risk groups and preventive strategies
* Evaluation of the clinical impact of the ADR on patients and on entire populations
* Providing information to health care providers and the patients
* Eventual regulation of drug use

Table 2. Sources of Information Available in Sweden for the Evaluation of Drug Safety

Type of Register	Year Started
ADVERSE DRUG REACTION ORIENTED	
Spontaneous ADR reports	1965
Intensive Hospital Monitoring	1979*
DRUG UTILIZATION ORIENTED	
County of Jämtland; individual prescriptions	1970
County of Tierp; individual prescriptions	1971
Total drug sales register	1972
Prescription Sample	1974
Diagnosis and Therapy Survey	1978
PATIENT AND DISEASE ORIENTED	
Causes of Death Register	1911
Cancer Register	1959
Birth Defects Register	1965
Hospital Discharge Diagnoses	1968
Medical Birth Records Register	1973

* only one limited study

For reports concerning serious reactions much emphasis is put on identifying the nature of the reaction and the clinical course thereof. Whenever there are nationally or internationally agreed criteria for reactions or drug-induced diseases we apply these, e.g., for hematological reactions[4], liver reactions[5] and some neurologic reactions.[6] In this process the important work done in France[7] is greatly appreciated.

For causality assessment no special algorithm is used routinely, but the following points are considered.

1. Is there a reasonable temporal connection between drug intake and the suspected reaction?
2. Is there a logical pharmacologic explanation for the reaction or has it been described before?
3. Does the reaction diminish or disappear when the dose of the drug is reduced or suspended?
4. Can the patient's primary disease elicit similar symptoms?
5. Can some other drug given cause the same symptom or can the symptom be an interaction?
6. Did the same symptom occur on previous exposures or did it recur on rechallenge?

A more detailed discussion on the important problem of causality assessment is presented in a separate chapter by Dr. Jones.

Since 1965 the reporting has slowly increased. In 1975, when the reporting of serious and new reactions was made mandatory for physicians and dentists, there was an increase in the reporting rate, but the trend was otherwise not much influenced. Since the mid 1980s reporting has levelled off at between 2,500 and 3,000 reports per year. On an international comparison this is relatively high but still it is clearly unsatisfactory, especially in comparison with the number of patients hospitalized because of adverse reactions.[8,9]

RESULTS OBTAINABLE BY ANALYZING REPORTS ALONE

A spontaneous reporting system can, in its basic form, be regarded as an incomplete (and at worst biased) case series, without any information on the size or characteristics of the population exposed to the drug except the indication for treatment. In those situations it is rarely possible to establish a causal connection between the adverse event and the drug from spontaneous reports, unless:

a) there is at least one case with a positive rechallenge and some other supportive cases without known confounding drugs or diseases, or
b) there is a cluster of exposed cases reported and the background incidence of the adverse event is close to zero, and there is no confounding.

Even though the reappearance of an adverse event when the drug is given again is no proof of causality[10], one can in practice be rather reassured that there is strong evidence for a causal connection if one has a cluster of cases with good clinical information, and where the same event has reappeared at least once in each patient. This is true if the event in question is of a type that should diminish or disappear after withdrawal of the drug and not reappear spontaneously. Thus, the observation of five cases of aseptic meningitis which reappeared within hours after taking the antibiotic trimethoprim for urinary tract infections[11], will convince most clinicians (and lawyers, if not philosophers) that this drug did and can cause such a reaction. For typical "hit and run" effects like thromboembolic diseases and for diseases which can be cyclic, information on rechallenge can, however, be misleading.

However, information on rechallenge is rare in most spontaneous reporting systems. In a study aimed at comparing the information in and evaluation of spontaneous reports from the Nordic countries, it was found that there was information on a positive re-exposure in only 13% of 200 consecutive non-fatal cases.[12]

A situation meeting the second criterion may be the one seen with the cardiovascular drug aprindine, where four to five cases of agranulocytosis reported in the Netherlands during the first two years on the market made a strong case for a causal relationship[13], as the background incidence of agranulocytosis is only 5 - 8 per million inhabitants per year.[4]

Usually drug profiles can be produced without knowledge of denominator data. The profiles of some nonsteroidal anti-inflammatory analgesics are shown in Figure 1.

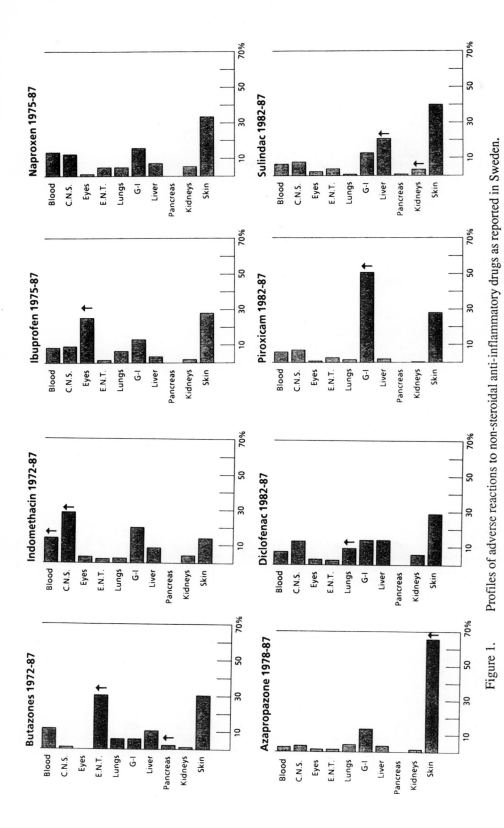

Figure 1. Profiles of adverse reactions to non-steroidal anti-inflammatory drugs as reported in Sweden.

The different appearance of these profiles indicates that the distribution of reported reactions certainly differs among these drugs. One must, however, be very cautious in the interpretation of such differences, since there are many sources of errors and bias that may be of importance. When looking at the butazones and ear, nose, and throat (ENT) reactions, we probably see a real difference, as the parotitis and salivary gland inflammations induced by these drugs almost never have been reported for other NSAIDs, except for sulindac. The high proportion of visual disturbances reported for ibuprofen may, on the other hand, be an example of selective reporting. At about the time ibuprofen was marketed in Sweden, there was an article suggesting that ibuprofen could induce optical neuritis, and that was widely discussed in Sweden. This led to an influx of reports of diffuse visual disturbances, but not one single well documented case of optical neuritis. It is also clear that, unless the total incidence of ADRs is equal, e.g., for ibuprofen and the butazones, the different proportions of specific ADRs, for example blood dyscrasias, cannot be interpreted as differences in risk. For such comparisons, estimates of the denominators are needed.

USE OF SPONTANEOUS REPORTING DATA FOR AGGREGATE ANALYSES

Additional Data Sources Used to Estimate Denominators and Disease Occurrence

Today many drug regulatory authorities and pharmaceutical manufacturers have access to information by which both the size and characteristics of the exposed population and the background incidence of diseases can be estimated. The sources available in Sweden are shown in Table 2.

In Sweden all pharmacies belong to one state owned corporation and the total amount of drugs delivered to different pharmacies since 1972 and hospitals since 1976, by region, are computerized and stored. The amounts sold can easily be calculated as number of packs, tablets, or so called defined daily doses (DDD).[14]

Since 1974 a random sample of 1/288 and since 1983 1/25 prescriptions has been selected in pharmacies. Information about the age and sex of the patient, and the name, amount, and daily prescribed dose of the drug is coded and computerized.

Since 1978 the Diagnosis and Therapy Survey has been run in collaboration with the pharmaceutical industry, the National Corporation of Pharmacies, the Medical Association, and the National Board of Health. In this survey a random sample of physicians each week register the indication for all drugs prescribed.

All this information is on an aggregate, non individual, basis. There is also a small individual prescription register in the county of Jämtland, where drug purchases for 1/7 of the population has been continuously recorded since 1970. Information from all these sources are published annually in a book, Swedish Drug Statistics.[15]

The morbidity and mortality oriented registers function in much the same way as in other countries. While the information in the cancer register, the malformation register, and the medical birth record register is of high quality, it is slow, with a backlog of one to three years. The information in the mortality register and hospital diagnosis register is produced more quickly but is sometimes less accurate.

Estimation of Reporting Rates

If the rate of reporting is known the estimate of the numerator becomes more accurate. From studies using registers of hospital discharge diagnoses it has been possible to calculate reporting rates for some areas, ADRs, and periods of time. In general between 20% and 40% of serious reactions such as blood dyscrasias, thromboembolic disease, and Stevens-Johnson syndrome, identified by checking medical records of patients discharged with these diagnoses, have been found to be reported in Sweden.[16] By checking all positive BCG cultures in bacteriologic laboratories, it was found that almost 80% of all children who developed an osteitis after BCG vaccination had been reported.[17] However, these reporting rates probably cannot be generalized. They are important to know when evaluating the data, but should not be used to correct for under-reporting in the calculations, as the reporting rate may well be drug-specific.

Identification of Mechanisms and Risk Groups

As soon as it has been established that a drug can induce a certain adverse reaction, it becomes very important to look for the mechanisms which could be involved and to try to identify if any special group of patients is at increased risk or if any measures could be taken to reduce the risk, either at a patient or a population level.

In this work usually a multitude of different methods must be applied, both in the laboratory and on a population level. Also in this work, a good spontaneous reporting system can be of value in certain circumstances, if the data can be compared to sales and prescription data or the patients can be subjected to special investigations.

In one study on the characteristics of patients developing hypoglycemia during treatment with glibenclamide (an oral antidiabetic drug), it was found that the distribution of prescribed daily doses in reports of severe hypoglycemic episodes was similar to that in the general population, but that patients hospitalized because of severe hypoglycemia were older. In addition, a previous episode of cerebrovascular disease seemed to be a risk factor for severe hypoglycemia.[18] In one of the first follow-up studies published on oral contraceptives and thromboembolic disease, it was found that women who were reported to have developed a deep vein thrombosis while taking oral contraceptives were of the blood group O more often than would have been expected from the distribution of blood groups in the population.[19] In a similar study[20] it was found that patients reported to have developed lupoid reactions while taking hydralazine for hypertension had a genetic defect in their capacity to acetylate the drug (slow acetylators) in a much higher percentage than was expected from the distribution in the population of this phenotype. Finally some years after the antidiabetic drug phenformin had been taken off the market because of its high risk for eliciting a serious metabolic adverse effect, lactic acidosis, it was reported that the metabolism of phenformin had polymorphic distribution in the population that co-varied with that of debrisoquine.[21] The authors proposed that slow metabolizers of phenformin were at increased risk for developing lactic acidosis, implying that the drug could be used if patients were tested for this enzyme deficiency. We did a follow-up study on patients who survived an episode of lactic acidosis while taking phenformin.[22] Out of seven cases only one was a slow metabolizer which is consistent with the normal frequency of 8% slow metabolizers. The study was too small to investigate if slow metabolizers really were at increased risk, but the main conclusion was that this genetic trait was not a prerequisite for developing the reaction and, therefore, the drug could not be safely reintroduced with patients tested before starting therapy.

Estimation of Incidence Rate, Rate Ratio, and Rate Difference

If information from an efficient spontaneous reporting system can be combined with drug sales and prescription statistics, it is often possible to derive a rough estimate of the frequency or incidence rate of an ADR. Such estimates can, of course, never reach the accuracy of those derived from clinical trials or formal epidemiological PMS studies. However, they can serve as a first indicator of the size of a potential problem and for very rare reactions they may actually be the only conceivable measure.

With knowledge of the number of DDDs sold and the average prescribed daily dose (PDD), it is possible to get a rough estimate of the total person time of exposure for a particular drug.

If prescription statistics are available, the number of cases reported per prescription may actually be a better estimate of the risk among outpatients than if the number of treatment weeks are calculated from sales data, at least for antibiotics where doses and treatment times may vary with patient age and indication.

For example, in Sweden the frequency of reports of serum-sickness like reactions and erythema multiforme among children aged 0 to 9 years prescribed cephaclor (an antibiotic) as a suspension, were 17 and 4 per 10,000 prescriptions, respectively, while no such reactions were reported among adults using tablets. These results could imply that there is something wrong with the mixture (e.g., a stability problem) which causes the reactions. Age-dependent differences in reporting or in actual immunological reactivity are, however, other possible explanations, and one must always be extremely careful in the interpretation of such data.

If the background incidence of a disease is known or can be estimated from other sources, it is sometimes possible to get rough estimates of rate ratios and rate differences from spontaneously reported data on ADRs and sales and prescription statistics. This technique was first applied in 1983 when we investigated a possible relationship between a new antidepressant drug and the development of Guillain-Barré syndromes in patients experiencing flu-like hypersensitivity reactions from this new medicine.[23]

Examples

A series of examples of risk estimates of drug-induced blood dyscrasias will be used here to illustrate how the use of such data have developed in Sweden.

Acetazolamide associated aplastic anemia. Single cases of aplastic anemia developing in patients taking acetazolamide (a carbonic anhydrase inhibiting diuretic drug which is used mainly for the treatment of glaucoma) have been reported since the drug was introduced in the mid-1950s.[24] There are no estimates of the incidence of this reaction, but it was generally thought that it was very rare and certainly occurred less often than with chloramphenicol. Through a careful investigation of the cases reported in relation to sales and prescription data and with knowledge of the total incidence of aplastic anemia, we found some evidence that this reaction was much more common than hitherto appreciated.

Pancytopenia was defined as the occurrence in peripheral blood of hemoglobin <100 g/l, total white cell count <3.5 x 10^9/l, and thrombocytes <50 x 10^9/l. There should be no signs of hemolysis or acute bleeding nor of intravascular coagulation. Patients receiving cytostatic or immunosuppressive drug treatment or radiation treatment within three months were excluded. Aplastic anemia was defined as pancytopenia with a clearly hypoplastic bone marrow. There should be no signs of granulomatous disease or malignancy in the bone marrow.

Between 1972 and 1988, 11 cases of aplastic anemia were reported to have occurred in exposed patients in Sweden.[25] Based on sales and prescription data it could be estimated that the total exposure time was 195,400 patient-years during the same period of time, giving a reported incidence of about one in 18,000 patient-years (Figure 2). From a population-based case-control study of aplastic anemia in which Sweden participated[26], it could be estimated that the total yearly incidence of aplastic anemia in the relevant age groups was 3.2 and 6.3 per million inhabitants among men and women respectively.

In the case-control study it was not possible to estimate the rate ratio for the association between acetazolamide and aplastic anemia, because there were no exposed controls. If the spontaneously reported incidence of aplastic anemia among people

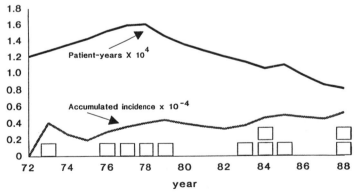

Figure 2. Use of acetazolamide in Sweden 1972-1988 and number of reported patients developing aplastic anemia. Solid line shows the number of patient years of exposure based on sales data. Hatched line represents the cumulative incidence per 10,000 patient-years. Each box represents one case of aplastic anemia.

exposed to acetazolamide is compared with the total incidence of aplastic anemia from the case-control study, the rate ratio could be estimated to be 13 (95% confidence intervals 9-25). It was 25 (95% confidence intervals 9-67) for men and 10 (95% confidence intervals 4-23) for women.

Several potential sources of errors in this study must be recognized. The degree of under-reporting in this actual case is unknown, but in one study[27] the reporting rate for aplastic anemia was found to be 30%. Since then reporting in general has doubled. There is no known association between glaucoma and aplastic anemia which could act as a confounder, but some of these patients had taken other drugs during the last six months before the detection of their aplastic anemia. In this case there were only two patients who had been treated with drugs which on clinical pharmacological grounds seem to be reasonable alternatives, but it is a clear limitation that multiple drug exposures cannot be corrected for in a rough analysis such as this.

Nine of the 11 cases of aplastic anemia developed during the first three months of treatment which, as in the study of zimeldine-associated Guillian-Barré Syndrome, indicated that the risk was not independent of time. If so, the traditional way of expressing risk as the number of cases per person-time of exposure would be a crude average with limited clinical value.

In a further study of the risk of developing agranulocytosis from the use of dapsone in the treatment of dermatitis herpetiformis, we could examine this more closely. The seven cases reported between 1972 - 1988 represented 1 case per 3000 patient-years of treatment.[28] With knowledge of the total incidence of agranulocytosis the relative risk could be estimated to be 50 (Table 3) and the excess risk to be 1/3000 patient-years. However, the total incidence of the disease, dermatitis herpetiformis, was only 11 cases per million inhabitants per year and, therefore, not more than about 1700 new cases had appeared during the study period. As all new cases are started on dapsone and the reaction almost always develops during the first months of treatment, these 1700 cases form a clinically more relevant denominator. The seven cases of agranulocytosis then represented a risk of about 1/250 - 1/500 patients depending on whether cases taking other suspected drugs were included or excluded. These latter risk estimates clearly differ from the traditional 1/3000 patient-years, and the difference is large enough to infer differences in the strategy for following patients with regard to routine monitoring of blood counts. However, as dapsone is more or less the only available drug treatment for dermatitis herpetiformis, even a risk of this magnitude is most probably acceptable. In a further study[29] it has been possible to carry the analysis a step further and evaluate the risk during different periods of treatment.

Sulfasalazine associated agranulocytosis. During the period 1972 through 1989, 60 outpatients were reported to have developed agranulocytosis fulfilling internationally accepted criteria[4]. The frequency of outpatient agranulocytosis could be calculated to

Table 3.   Dapsone Associated Agranulocytosis

Total incidence	6.7/million per year
Total person time	137,340,000
Total No. of cases	920
Exposed cases	7
Person time among exposed	21,300 years
Incidence among exposed	0.00033/year
	1/3,000 years
Non-exposed cases	913
Person time unexposed	137,320,000
Incidence among unexposed	0.000006648/year

$$RR = \frac{0.00033}{0.000006648} = 50$$

95% confidence interval 21-130

1.1/million DDD, which equals 1 case in about 1800 patient-years when the PDD is taken into account.   Again the cases were very unevenly distributed in time, as 14 developed agranulocytosis within the first 30 days of treatment, 44 between days 31-90, and only 2 cases appeared between day 91 - 365.
      In order to estimate the risk of agranulocytosis during different treatment periods, it is mandatory to have data on individual treatment times for all those treated. This does not exist outside a prescription register and we do not have that in Sweden yet. However, there has been a prescription register covering 1/7 of the population in one county since 1970, the county of Jämtland. In this prescription register there was information on the actual prescribing to and purchasing of sulfasalazine for all 173 patients who had ever been prescribed this drug. The average age and sex distribution of these patients was similar to that in all of Sweden (as assessed from the prescription survey). Also the average prescribed daily dose in the county of Jämtland was similar to that in all of Sweden. We therefore felt comfortable with the assumption that the treatment times in Jämtland would be representative of those in all of Sweden. Using this assumption it was then possible to calculate:

> 1) The number of patients in all of Sweden that were
>   represented by the total number of PDDs sold.
> 2) The distribution of treatment times in this cohort.

      The distribution of treatment times and the risk estimates are depicted in Figure 3. From the figure it can be seen how the risk increases to as much as 1/700 patients between day 31 and 90, whereafter it almost disappears.
      The results of this study clearly indicate the importance of taking time into account in the risk expression and preferably the risk should be presented as some kind of hazard function when dealing with idiosyncratic reactions.   Carson, Strom et al did something similar when studying the risk of gastrointestinal bleeding from non-steroidal anti-inflammatory analgesics[30], but otherwise this approach has rarely if at all been used in pharmacoepidemiology.

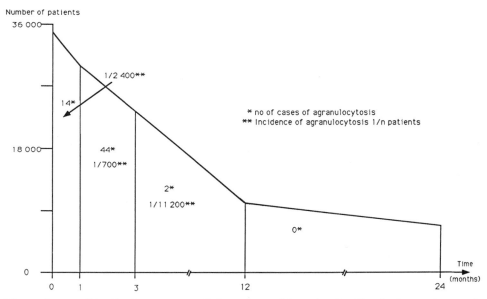

Figure 3.   Distribution pattern of the estimated length of sulfasalazine treatment in 34,500 patients, and the length of treatment until diagnosis of agranulocytosis in 60 patients.   The incidence of agranulocytosis estimated during 1 month, and 3-12 months of sulfasalazine therapy.

Spontaneous reporting is recognized as the most effective method to discover rare but serious adverse reactions. It is, however, not thought to yield valid estimates of frequency or risk. This is also probably most often the case, especially when considering drug-related beneficial or adverse effects concerning cancer or in situations where the reaction under study is of type A, as these reactions most often are common. There are, however, situations where the reaction under study is rare and of type B and the background incidence of the disease is low, where it seems possible to obtain adequately valid data with the approach outlined in the examples above.

We have compared the risk estimates derived from our monitoring system with those from an international case-control study of blood dyscrasias in Table 4. The estimates of both relative and excess risks were similar enough that would have, most probably, led to the same clinical and regulatory evaluations of the problem for butazones, co-trimoxazole, and sulfasalazine.[4,31] For acetazolamide no estimate could be derived in the case-control study, because no controls were exposed.

Table 4.   Comparison of Risk Estimates of Sulfa-induced Agranulocytosis from the Swedish Drug Monitoring System and the International Agranulocytosis and Aplastic Anemia Study

| Source | Swedish Drug Monitoring | | Case Control Study | |
	Sulfasalazine	*TMS*	*Sulfasalazine*	*TMS*
	Swedish ADR register	Swedish ADR register	S-IAAAS	IAAAS
Time Period	1983-89	1976-85	1983-89	1980-86
No of exposed cases included	19	7	13	12
Relative risk	107	17	123	12
Excess risk (/million treatment days)	1.8	0.3	1.8	>1.6*

*   Exposure for 3 or more days
TMS = trimethoprim + sulfamethoxazole

CONCLUSION

It is proposed that adequately correct estimates can be obtained with a good monitoring system under the conditions outlined in Table 5. Apart from a high and preferably known reporting rate, it is important to know the background prevalence and incidence rate of the disease or event under study and to get good clinical data on the exposed cases in order to validate the diagnosis of the reported event. It must, however, be clearly stated that a spontaneous monitoring system is of little value in the quantification of associations between common adverse events and common exposures, e.g., the risk of gastrointestinal bleeding from aspirin and other non-steroidal anti-inflammatory drugs.

Table 5.	Suggested Characteristics of Situations Where a Good Spontaneous Reporting System Together with Sales, Prescription, and Morbidity Statistics Can Give Adequate Estimates of Risk

A drug	taken in standardized doses for long term treatment or defined short-term periods elicits
A reaction	which is serious and has a low background rate and few confounding conditions
Especially	
if	the relative risk (RR) is high and the reaction is well known

REFERENCES

1. G. R. Venning, Identifications of adverse reactions to new drugs, II - How were 18 important adverse reactions discovered and with what delay?, *BMJ*. 286:289-292 (1983).

2. B-E. Wiholm, Spontaneous reporting outside the USA, in: "Pharmacoepidemiology," B. Strom, ed., Churchville Livingstone, New York, 119-134 (1989).

3. I. R. Edwards, M. Lindquist, B-E Wiholm, and E. Napke, Quality criteria for early signals of possible adverse drug reactions, *Lancet*. II:156-58 (1990).

4. The International Agranulocytosis and Aplastic Anemia Study: Risk of agranulocytosis and aplastic anemia, A first report of their relation to drugs with special reference ta analgesics, *JAMA*. 256:1749-57 (1986).

5. C. Bénichou, and G. Danan, Criteria of drug-induced liver disorders. Report of an international consensus meeting, *J Hepatol*. (1990).

6. Diagnostic criterions for Guillain-Barré, National Institute for Neurological and Communicative Disorders and Stroke (NINCDS), *JAMA*. 249:1709-10 (1978).

7. G. Danan, Consensus meetings on causality assessment of drug-induced liver injury, *J Hepatol*. 7:132-36 (1988).

8. B. Beermann, G. Björck, and M. Groschinsky-Grind, Admissions to a medical clinic due to drugs and intoxications, *Läkartidningen*. 75:959-960 (1978).

9. U. Bergman, and B-E Wiholm, Drug-Related Problems Causing Admission to a Medical Clinic, *Eur J Clin Pharmacol*. 20:193-200 (1981).

10. K. J. Rothman, Causal inference in epidemiology, in: "Modern epidemiology," Boston, Little, Brown and Company, pp. 7-21 (1986).

11. J. Carlson and B-E Wiholm, Trimethoprim associated aseptic meningitis, *Scand J Infect Dis*. 19:687-691 (1987).

12. Nordic Council on Medicines, Drug Monitoring in the Nordic Countries, An evaluation of simimlarities and differences, NLN Publication No. 25, Nordic Council on Medicines, Uppsala, Sweden.

13. R. van Leeuwen, and R. H. B. Meyboom, Agranulocytosis and aprinidine, *Lancet*. II:1137 (1976).

14. Nordic Statistics on Medicines 1975-1977, Part II. Nordic Council on Medicines, Box 607, S-751 25 Uppsala, Sweden.

15. Statistisk sammanställning 1979-88 (Swedish Drug Statistics), "Introduction and codes in English," National Corporation of Swedish Pharmacies, S-105 14, Stockholm, Sweden.

16. B-E Wiholm, Spontaneous reporting of ADR. *in*: "Detection and prevention of adverse drug reactions," Skandia International Symposia, Almqvist & Wiksell Stockholm, p. 152-167 (1983).

17. M. Böttiger, V. Romanus, C. deVerdier, and G. Boman, Osteitis and other complications caused by generalized BCG-itis, Experiences in Sweden, *Acta Pediat Scand.* 71:471-478 (1982).

18. K. Asplund, and B-E Wiholm, Glibenclamide-associated hypoglycemia, a report on 57 cases, *Diabetologia* 24:412-417 (1983).

19. H. Jick, D. Slone, B. Westerholm, W. H. W. Inman, M. P. Vessey, S. Shapiro, G. P. Lewis, and J. Worcester, Venous thromboembolic disease and ABO blood type, *Lancet.* I:539-542 (1969).

20. I. Strandberg, G. Boman, L. Hassler, and F. Sjöqvist, Acetylaltor phenotype in patients with hydralazine-induced lupoid syndrome, *Acta Med Scand.* 200:267-371 (1976).

21. J. R. Idle, The various criteria in establishing polymorphism of drug oxidation, *in*: Workshop on polymorphism of drug oxidation in man, (Oct 11-12, 1980, Bonn).

22. B-E Wiholm, G. Alvan, L. Bertilsson, and et. al., Hydroxylation of Debrisoquine in Patients with Lactic Acidosis after Phenformin, *Lancet.* pp. 1099 (1981).

23. J. Fagius, P. O. Osterman, Å. Siden, and B-E Wiholm, Guillain-Barré Syndrome following zimeldine treatment, *J Neurol Neurosurg Psychiatry.* 48:65-69 (1985).

24. F. T. Fraunfelder, M. S. Meyer, G. C. Bagby Jr., and M. N. Dreis, Hematologic reactions to carbonic anhydrase inhibitors, *Am J Ophtalmol.* 100:79-81 (1985).

25. M. Keisu, B-E Wiholm, Å. Öst, Ö. Mortimer, Acetazolamide associated Aplastic Anemia, *J Intern Med.* (in press).

26. The International Agranulocytosis and Aplastic Anemia Study: Incidence of aplastic anemia, The relevance of diagnostic criteria, *Blood.* 70:1718-1721.

27. L. E. Böttiger, and B. Westerholm, Drug-induced blood-dyscrasias in Sweden, *Br Med J.* 3:339-343 (1973).

28. P. Hörnsten P, M. Keisu, and B-E Wiholm, The Incidence of Agranulocytosis During Treatment of Dermatitis Herpetiformis With Dapsone as Reported in Sweden 1972-1988, *Arch Dermatol.* 26:919-922 (1990).

29. M. Keisu, and E. Ekman, Sulfasalazine associated agranulocytosis in Sweden 1972-1989, Clinical features, and estimation of its incidence, *European J Clin Pharmacol.* (in press).

30. J. L. Carson, B. L. Strom, K. A. Soper, S. L. West, M. L. Morse, The association of nonsteroidal anti-inflammatory drugs with upper gastrointestinal tract bleeding, *Arch Intern Med.* 147:1054-9 (1987).

31. M. Keisu, E. Ekman, and B-E Wiholm, Comparing risk estimates of sulfa induced agranulocytosis from the Swedish Drug Monitoring System and a case-control study, *Eur J Clin Pharmacol.* (in press).

SPONTANEOUS MONITORING OF ADVERSE REACTIONS TO DRUGS,

PROCEDURES, AND EXPERIENCES IN THE NETHERLANDS

R. H. B. Meyboom, M.D.

Netherlands Centre for Monitoring of
Adverse Reactions to Drugs
Rijswijk, The Netherlands

INTRODUCTION

In the sixties, after the tragic epidemic of malformed children born to mothers who had used thalidomide during pregnancy, in many countries throughout the world a start was made with monitoring of the safety of medicines. The thalidomide disaster had shown the community at large that medicines can be an unexpected and unpredictable cause of serious adverse reactions and that, when a drug is widely used, the number of victims may be large. It established the understanding that new medicines must be monitored for their safety after introduction. The thalidomide case was, however, not an isolated experience, but one in a series of outbreaks of more or less serious drug-induced disorders. Table 1 gives a list of examples of such disorders that have occurred in the past 100 years. Every example has its own story and lesson. Some cases have been very sad, but nevertheless received little public attention (e.g., malignant disorders as a late complication of the once widely used contrast medium thorium dioxide). The examples in the table also show the great diversity of drug-induced pathology (including blood dyscrasias, hepatitis, renal failure, polyneuropathy, deafness, psychosis, malformations, or cancer), which practically encompasses the entire spectrum of human diseases. This series has continued up to the present time, despite modern drug regulation and monitoring. Apparently it is inevitable that occasionally more or less serious adverse reactions come to light only after a drug has been marketed and has come into general use.

Several factors may be responsible for this situation. Of special importance is that the usual clinical trials are much better suited for the assessment of efficacy rather than safety. As compared with the use of a drug after introduction for general use, clinical trials include small numbers of (highly) selected patients and are of relatively short duration. Furthermore, the parameters to be measured or monitored are fixed and limited in number. In other words, the conditions of a clinical trial are very different from those in "real life," and at the time of marketing the knowledge about a drug is more or less incomplete, especially with regard to less frequent possible adverse reactions.

In this light it is a somewhat paradoxical situation that, as soon as a new drug is approved by the registration authority, it is considered to be an established treatment and so may - wrongly - lose much of its experimental character.

The study of the safety of medicines, in qualitative and quantitative respects, faces many methodological, ethical, and financial problems. Up to the present time, our knowledge of adverse reactions to drugs is, to a large extent, based on anecdotal descriptions of practical experiences in the medical literature and - especially in the past 15 years - on the contributions by country-wide voluntary reporting systems. This knowledge accumulates only gradually during the years, or even decades, after the

Drug Epidemiology and Post-Marketing Surveillance, Edited by B.L. Strom
and G. Velo, Plenum Press, New York, 1992

Table 1.   Review of Serious Drug-Induced Diseases in the Past 100 Years

1880*	Chloroform	Cardiac arrest
1923	Cinchophen	Hepatitis
1933	Aminophenazone	Agranulocytosis
1938	Sulfanilamide (diethylene glycol)	Fatal poisoning
1946	Streptomycine	Deafness
1950	Thorium dioxide	Malignant disorders
1952	Chloramphenicol	Aplastic anemia
1953	Phenacetin	Nephropathy
1954	Stalinon	Fatal poisoning
1958	Isoniazid	Hepatitis
1961	Thalidomide	Phocomelia
1966	Oral contraceptives	Thromboembolic disease
1967	Sympathomimetics	Asthma deaths
1969	Aminorex	Pulmonary hypertension
1970	Clioquinol	Myelo-optic neuropathy
	Nitrofurantoin	Neuropathy; pneumonitis
	Phenacetin	Urinary tract carcinoma
1972	Diethylstilbestrol	Vaginal carcinoma; urogenital malformations
	Bismuth	Encephalopathy
1973	Neuroleptics	Tardive dyskinesia
1974	Practolol	Sclerosing peritonitis
	Clindamycin	Pseudomembranous colitis
1975	Clozapine	Agranulocytosis
	Venopyronum	SLE syndrome
1976	Glafenine	Anaphylaxis
1979	Triazolam	Psychosis; amnesia
1980	Tielenic acid	Liver & kidney injury
1982	Benoxaprofen	Photodermatitis
1981	Ketoconazole	Hepatitis
1983	Zimeldine	Polyradiculoneuritis
	Osmosin	Distal intestinal ulcers
	Zomepirac	Anaphylaxis
1985	Cianidanol	Hepatitis; hemolysis
	Mianserine	Agranulocytosis
1986	Nomifensine	Fever, hepatitis, hemolytic anemia
1986	Almitrine	Polyneuropathy
1987	Ofloxacin	Psychosis; hypersensitivity
1987	Suprofen	Renal injury
	Isoxicam	Toxic epidermal necrolysis
1990	Pirprofen	Hepatitis

* The dates refer to either the discovery of the adverse reaction or to the time measures were taken

introduction of a drug. Especially in the past few years, with the development of pharmacoepidemiology, and thanks to the work of outstanding institutions such as the Drug Safety Research Unit in Southampton, there is an increasing understanding of this complex subject matter and the possible techniques enabling the exact measurement of the safety of different medicines.

In a modern society new drugs should only be introduced into human medicine in the presence of an appropriate safety monitoring system. The first step in this respect usually is the establishment of a country-wide case reporting system, often referred to as

"Spontaneous Monitoring" or "Voluntary Reporting" (VR). The basic elements of such a national system have been outlined in a WHO Technical Report in 1972.[1] Since then information on VR in various countries has been presented at several occasions, disclosing considerable differences in procedures and attitudes.[2-6] A detailed account of VR in the United Kingdom has recently been given by Rawlins.[7] The present article reviews the experiences with VR in the Netherlands.

ABOUT ADVERSE DRUG REACTIONS

The actions of most drugs are more or less non-selective. In other words, the therapeutic effect is usually associated with side effects, or - at least - the risk thereof. Because of their heterogeneity and multiplicity, side effects and adverse reactions are difficult to classify. On practical grounds, a classification can be made as is presented in Table 2. Side effects resulting directly from the pharmacological actions of a drug can be accurately studied in clinical trials, and their frequencies and severity with different doses are usually well known at the time of marketing of the drug. Serious adverse reactions, on the other hand, usually occur in only a minority of patients. Apparently such patients have certain predisposing conditions, such as immunologic or metabolic abnormalities, but often these factors are only poorly understood.

Adverse reactions may show a remarkable absence of a dose relationship, and are notoriously difficult to reproduce and study in experimental conditions. Adverse responses may also follow interactions between medicines or with drugs of other origin (e.g., alcohol, stimulants, foods). Furthermore, special situations may introduce special problems, such as maternal drug use resulting in prenatal exposure, or drug use in hemodialysis patients.

From the point of view of drug monitoring, the WHO has proposed a very broad definition of an adverse drug reaction, including any response that is "noxious, is unintended and occurs at doses normally used in man".[1] This definition essentially distinguishes an adverse reaction from an overt overdose (intoxication).

For various reasons, the "frequency" of adverse reactions in general, in other words the proportion of human diseases which is drug-induced, is very difficult to calculate. Adverse reactions are reported to be responsible for approximately 2 - 6% of admissions to hospital medical wards and to occur in about 20% of hospitalized patients.[8] The frequency of adverse reactions is mainly determined by the number and nature of drugs used and, indirectly, by the diseases of the patients.[9] The frequence of adverse reactions in a medical ward strongly increases when hematological (leukemia, lymphoma) or oncologic patients are included. Important adverse reactions, on the other hand, such as gastrointestinal hemorrhage or perforation, may escape statistics, since these patients are often admitted directly to a surgical ward.

The more seriously ill a patient is, the higher is his or her chance of experiencing an adverse event, but also of receiving toxic drugs. In other words, a large proportion of severely ill patients (including cardiovascular, oncologic, or infectious diseases) experience unpleasant or life-threatening adverse events, but the differentiation from the underlying diseases is often difficult. Since the frequency of adverse drug reactions "in general" is almost impossible to measure, quantitative studies should preferably focus on specific groups of drugs and patients.

AIMS AND PROCEDURES OF SPONTANEOUS MONITORING; EXPERIENCES IN THE NETHERLANDS

Voluntary Reporting System in the Netherlands

The Netherlands are only a small country, but with 14.5 million the number of inhabitants is larger than might be expected. There are about 35,800 medical doctors, including 6400 general practitioners and 12,000 specialists. There are only about 1400 pharmacies, but about 900 general practitioners provide independent pharmaceutical services and self-medication drugs are sold in a large number of chemist's shops.

The Netherlands Centre for Monitoring of Adverse Drug Reactions (NARD)[10] was established 25 years ago, as an initiative of the Royal Medical Association. The

Table 2.	Classification of Adverse Reactions
DRUG ACTIONS	Pharmacological effects, more frequent with high doses, can be reproduced and studied experimentally
PATIENT REACTIONS	Rare, occur only in hypersensitive patients (immuno-allergic, metabolic intolerance, idiosyncrasy), no clear dose relationship, can usually not be reproduced experimentally
DRUG INTERACTIONS	Interactions with other medicines, stimulants, foods or environmental drugs

NARD is now part of the Ministry of Welfare, Health and Culture in Rijswijk. Its main purpose was originally the prevention of future disasters, such as with thalidomide. The country-wide voluntary reporting system is, up to the present day, the most important source of information to the center. The experiences in the Netherlands have shown that VR is especially helpful for the following purposes:

- early detection of unknown adverse reactions,
- assessment of mechanisms and clinico-pathological characteristics of adverse reactions, and
- signalling of special problems.

The ultimate goal of a national adverse reactions monitoring center is the improvement of the safe use of medicines.

The procedures involved in VR and the assessment of the case reports at the NARD can be summarized as follows. In this context it is important to emphasize that a case report is not the simple registration of a drug effect, but is defined as "a notification by a physician concerning a patient with a disorder which is suspected to be drug-related, and is reported voluntarily and confidentially."

On receipt, each individual report is reviewed with regard to the source (registered physician?) and documentation (completeness of the data, follow-up?). Subsequently the relevance of the report is taken into consideration (whether the adverse reaction is new, serious, or otherwise unusual) and attention is paid to the possible pharmacological and pathological processes involved in its development. These considerations are followed by a preliminary assessment, in a systematic way, of the likelihood of a causal relationship between the drug and the adverse event (imputation; Table 3).

The next and very important step is that the reports are studied in interrelationship. By studying all reported suspected reactions to various drugs, clusters of interesting new suspected drug-reaction associations may be found. By comparing the patterns of events reported in association with different drugs, taking into account pharmacological, pathological, and epidemiological considerations, signals may be identified which are interesting and deserve further attention. At the same time, great care is taken to ensure that false signals are recognized as such and that they do not lead to premature publicity or action. Case reports usually concern suspicions rather than facts; great care is therefore needed in their interpretation. The NARD therefore has the support of a multidisciplinary scientific committee, for advising and taking responsibility with regard to the interpretation of the data and the scientific and public health implications of the reports. As will be discussed later on, many signals produced by VR need further investigation, for testing and clarification.

In view of the aims of VR, as already mentioned, reporting is needed of:

- all (suspected) adverse reactions to new drugs,
- all serious or unusual (suspected) reactions (i.e., also known reactions to "old" drugs),
- all reactions with a proven drug-disease relationship.

Table 3.   Causality Terms as Used by the NARD

1	Unclassified	incomplete or conflicting data; time relation unclear (e.g., carcinogenesis)
2	Unlikely	time relation seems inappropriate; other cause more likely

Only when the time relation is compatible:

3	Possible	relationship uncertain but not impossible; may be coincidence; as 4 but with fewer details
4	Probable	available evidence consistent with a reaction to the suspected drug; no likely alternative; no definite proof; as 5 but with fewer details
5	Certain	well documented case, all evidence implicates the drug; alternatives ruled out

The reasons for suspecting a disorder to be drug related are usually based on one or more of the following considerations: the time association between the drug and the event, the pharmacological plausability, and the absence of any other obvious explanation. Also, the localization of a reaction (e.g., contact dermatitis) may draw attention to a drug. VR is mainly focused on disorders which have characteristic features and a low spontaneous frequency of occurrence. The method is less suitable for the study of nonspecific complaints and common symptoms, or of reactions that have no noticable time relationship with the use of a drug (e.g., long-term effects). Such events need other methods of study, including appropriate controls.

Detection of Adverse Reactions

A population of about 14.5 million inhabitants may be ideal for VR. With much smaller populations the number of users of any particular drug is likely to be too low for an early warning, whereas in very large countries, on the other hand, large numbers of case reports may become difficult to handle. In the past ten years, the NARD has received an annual number of case reports of only about 1000; the issue of underreporting is discussed below.

Signal generation by VR has a simple principle, in that a valuable signal may arise when different doctors throughout the country independently report the same unknown and unexpected adverse experiences with a drug. As soon as a signal is received, important further questions arise, with regard to confirmation and clarification: is the suspected reaction a genuine phenomenon (signal testing)?, how frequent is the reaction?, which processes are involved? and how can the reaction be prevented (risk factors)? Usually further investigations and other methods (epidemiological, pharmacological) are needed to provide these answers.

As a preliminary test it can be very helpful to compare the data with those in other countries and to ascertain whether a signal is supported by similar experiences reported to other national center. International communication is facilitated by the work of the WHO Collaborating Centre for International Drug Monitoring in Uppsala.[11]

Table 4 lists examples of adverse drug reactions which have been assessed in an early stage by the NARD, with the help of VR.[12-47] As the table shows, a wide variety of different disorders have been involved, with a predominance of hypersensitivity reactions such as skin reactions, blood disorders, hepatitis, and anaphylaxis, but also including, for example, psychiatric symptoms or biliary colic.

25

Table 4.   Examples of Adverse Reactions that were Reported in an Early Stage to the NARD

Glafenine	Anaphylactic shock
Benzydamine	Visual & psychic effects
Practolol	Oculomucocutaneous syndrome
Aprindine	Agranulocytosis
Metrizamide / iopamidol	Aseptic meningitis
Triazolam	Psychosis, amnesia
Nomifensine	Fever, hepatitis
Camazepam	Rash
Cimetidine	Interstitial nephritis
Ticlopidine	Granulocytopenia, Thrombocytopenia
Ketoconazole	Hepatitis, anaphylaxis
Pinaverium bromide	Oesophagitis
Mianserine	Thrombocytopenia
Ketamine	Apnea
Mazindol	Testis pain
Scopolamine TTS	Delayed paradoxical effects
Pirenzepine	Granulocytopenia, Thrombocytopenia
Pirprofen	Hepatitis
Captopril / enalapril	Cough
Captopril	Gynecomastia
Terfenadine	Rash
Flunarizine	Depression, dyskinesia
Mebendazol	Hypersensitivity reactions
Labetotol	Fever
Isoflurane	Anaphylaxis
Indapamide	Rash, fever
Augmentin	Cholestatic hepatitis
Cinoxacin	Anaphylaxis
Fumaric acid-esters	Renal failure
Ceftriaxone	Biliary colics
Budesonide	Psychic reactions
Flutamide	Hepatitis
Naproxen	Interruption of menstruation

Although some of these associations have not yet been confirmed by other studies, the NARD has so far never issued a false signal, with the possible exception of obliterating bronchiolitis presumably spuriously associated with penicillamine.

Interactions have also been detected, especially those involving oral anticoagulants and contraceptives, and occasionally congenital malformations have been studied (Table 5;[48-56]).

Adverse reactions may not only be detected with new drugs, but - this needs to be emphasized - also with drugs which have already been in use for many years or even decades. Examples of such reactions are given in Table 6[(57-71)].

Many reactions have only very occasionally been described in the literature and knowledge of their characteristics have remained sparse. In such situations the practical experiences collected by VR may provide valuable additional information. Examples are visual effects of benzydamine[13], necrosis after phenylbutazone injections[72], pancreatitis induced by methyldopa[73] and, more recently, acute dystonic reactions in children elicited by domperidone.[74]

Adverse reactions are not only detected, but are sometimes also forgotten. Acute painful phlebitis as a side effect of ergotamine, for example, is mentioned in early volumes of Side Effects of Drugs, but has been omitted from later editions. The reports

Table 5.   Drug Interactions and Congenital Malformations Reported to the NARD

Azapropazone, Flurbiprofen, Amiodarone	-	Potentiation of coumarins
Modifast*	-	Inhibition of coumarins
Anticonvulsants, Griseofulvin	-	Inhibition of oral contraceptives
Ketoconazole	-	Alcohol intolerance
Coumarins	-	Face & bone malformations
Valproate	-	Spina bifida

* a slimming product containing vitamin K

Table 6.   New Adverse Reactions to Established Products, Reported to the NARD

Phenprocoumon	Hepatitis
Tetracycline	Esophageal ulcers
Glafenine	Hepatitis
Sulfasalazine	Male infertility
Nalidixic acid	Thrombocytopenia
Azapropazone	Photosensitivity
Spironolactone	Granulocytopenia
Oxolamine	Hallucinations
Nitrofurantoin	Parotitis
Valproate	Adult hyperammonemia
Paracetamol	Acute hypersensitivity
Amiodarone	Optic neuropathy
Oral contraceptives	Temperature elevation

to the NARD show beyond doubt, however, that these reactions do really occur in practice.[75]

As has been pointed out before, it can be very helpful to compare a signal, as a preliminary test, with the experiences in other countries. Close collaboration therefore exists between the NARD and monitoring centers in many different countries. The examples in Table 7 refer to issues which have been studied in collaboration with national centers in other countries and with the WHO Centre.

Detailed Analysis and Serial Assessment

The detailed assessment of reported cases can yield valuable additional information, sometimes with only small numbers. Observations in a single patient, for example, with a relapse on rechallenge, has recently provided strong evidence that clavulanic acid, in combination with amoxicillin, can cause cholestatic hepatitis.[40] In this case a new adverse reaction was detected on the basis of a single patient. The existence of this reaction has later been confirmed by similar reports, within and outside the Netherlands.[76]   Another example concerns propylthiouracil-induced agranulocytosis.[77] Although this is a well known complication, with an unusually high frequency of 1 in about 500 patients, little is known of the pathogenetic mechanism. Studies in one patient revealed immunological abnormalities. Autoimmune antibodies were found against membrane antigens of mature peripheral granulocytes, albeit weak. When granulocyte precursor cells (extracted from the bone marrow) were incubated with

27

Table 7.   Adverse Reactions Investigated by International Collaboration

Amiodarone	Optic neuropathy
Azapropazone	Photosensitivity
Griseofulvine	Interaction contraceptives
Indapamide	Rash, fever
Ketoconazole	Hepatitis
Mazindol	Testis pain
Nitrofurantoin	Hepatitis
Oxolamine	Hallucinations
Paracetamol	Acute hypersensitivity
Pirprofen	Hepatitis
Terfenadine	Rash
Cinoxacin	Anaphylaxis

PTU and subsequently cultured in the presence of recovery serum, there was a strong inhibition of colony forming units.   Interestingly, a similar effect was found for erythrocyte precursor cells. Without preincubation with PTU, on the other hand, no inhibition was found. It was concluded that, if this patient with agranulocytosis had continued to use PTU, general bone marrow depression with aplastic anemia would probably have developed. Furthermore, the findings illustrated that adverse reactions may be complex phenomena, and that the idea of "one drug one antigen" is an oversimplication. Other case-studies providing evidence of drug-dependent antibodies included thrombocytopenia associated with ticlopidine[22] and with mianserine.[26]

It is an important aspect of VR to try in an early stage to test a signal, for confirmation or refutation. A very interesting approach, which is sometimes possible, is to rechallenge the reported patients themselves, after invitation via their family doctors. In three patients with suspected paracetamol-induced methemoglobinemia, for example, no abnormal hemoglobins could be detected after rechallenge with paracetamol. Another interesting experience in this respect refers to terfenadine, an antihistamine drug considered to have no sedative effect and promoted for use by car drivers. The receipt of 20 case reports of profound sedation during the first few days of use of terfenadine, prompted the hypothesis that there might exist a subgroup of highly sensitive patients. When 10 of these patients volunteered for a comprehensive and controlled test, sedation could not be demonstrated, and it was concluded that terfenadine, at least under the conditions of the experiment - i.e., short-term use of a daily dose of 120 mg - probably does not cause sedation.[78] A case report of aplasia cutis in association with maternal use of methimazole initiated a restrospective survey in collaboration with the Amsterdam University Hospital. Although aplasia cutis is considered to be a "known" complication of antithyroid drugs, no such association was found in this study.[79] In a survey with the help of the Foundation of Health Care Information, Reye's Syndrome was found to be an extremely rare disorder in the Netherlands[80], and acetylsalicylic acid does not, in this respect, seem to be a very dangerous drug in our country.

Occasionally positive findings are reported which may have pharmacotherapeutic value. An example concerns a patient with known G6PD deficiency, who did not show signs of hemolysis during treatment with metronidazole, showing that this drug is probably safe in patients with G6PD deficiency.[81]

Country-wide VR provides a unique opportunity for collecting comparatively large series of patients with rare adverse reactions. The uniform "in depth" assessment of these cases can substantially increase our knowledge of the clinical and pathological features of adverse drug reactions. This in turn is helpful in facilitating the diagnosis in future patients.

The value of serial assessment can be illustrated by the NARD's recent studies on hepatic injury associated with the use of glafenine, nitrofurantoin, and ketoconazole. The study on glafenine included 27 reported patients with hepatic injury possibly or probably induced by this drug.[82] At that time only eight such cases had been described in the literature. The injury was predominantly hepatocellular in nature and was associated with jaundice in 75% of the patients; 25% had eosinophilia. There was a high case-fatality rate of 42%. These findings were very different as compared with liver damage associated with, for example, salicylates or phenylbutazone.

Nitrofurantoin and the closely related nifurtoinol are well known causes of hepatitis. A total of 53 patients have so far been described in 35 articles. The majority of cases concern chronic active hepatitis and, with a predominance of women in their fifties and a high frequency of autoimmune antibodies, the picture is very similar to that of chronic active autoimmune hepatitis. In a further 38 cases collected by VR by the NARD[83], however, a rather different picture emerged. There was a predominance of acute hepatitis, whereas the patients with chronic hepatitis were much older (which could not be explained by prescription figures). In the literature there is a correlation between autoimmune chronic active hepatitis and the HLA antigens B8 and DRW3, and between nitrofurantoin-associated chronic hepatitis and the antigen B8. When the HLA antigens were assessed in 9 of the 13 chronic hepatitis cases in the NARD series, however, no significant predominance of a particular haplotype was found.

The third study concerned a more recent subject: ketoconazole related hepatic injury.[84] At the time of the study, 16 such patients had been described in various anecdotal reports in the literature; one other study, including 33 cases, was based on VR in the United States.[85] When the NARD compared the findings in 50 patients with possible or probable ketoconazole-induced hepatic damage with the anecdotal cases, a lower fatality rate (0% versus 19%) and a different clinical spectrum were found. There was, on the other hand, a consistent similarity between the experiences as reported in the Netherlands and two studies based on VR in the United States[85] and the United Kingdom[86] (the latter covering 64 patients).

The systematic and detailed analysis of cases collected by VR presumably yields a more reliable picture of the characteristics of adverse reactions, as compared with that arising from anecdotal reporting in the literature.

Several studies by other centers on, for example, neurologic disturbances (polyradiculoneuritis induced by zimeldine) or hematologic disorders (nomifensin-induced hemolytic anemia[87]), have shown that other organ-systems can be studied in the same way.

Of importance for serial assessment are the requirements that reactions are reported at an early stage, to enable uniform assessment, that also "known" adverse reactions are reported, and that cases with a proven relationship with the drugs are reported. The latter may help to overcome the well known weakness of VR, that so often the relationship with the drug is a mere suspicion.

Signalling of Special Problems

The signalling of special problems with drugs and the identification of the most frequently reported causes of particular adverse reactions, is undoubtedly the most controversial use of VR. These matters are very important in social and regulatory respects and a very high level of scientific evidence is needed for responsible desicion making; evidence which may often not be solely provided by VR. It is especially in these situations that the dilemma is likely to arise that only formal - but time and money consuming - scientific studies can remove doubts and establish the exact frequencies of the reactions, whereas regulatory authorities are pressed to make decisions within a short time and with small budgets. One should always bear in mind, however, that VR is a method for problem signalling and not for problem solving.

Examples of problems which have in the past attracted the attention of the NARD (Table 8) are granulocytopenia reported in association with metamizole and other pyrazole derivatives[88], psychotic states with triazolam[10,89] and anaphylactic reactions after taking glafenine.[90]

Adverse Reactions in Children

Certain subgroups of patients, such as children or elderly people, are often not included in clinical trials. Postmarketing surveillance should therefore pay special attention to possible problems and risks in these groups. In a review of 11,542 case reports to the NARD of suspected adverse drug reactions, 521 (4.5%) were found to refer to patients of 14 years and younger.[91] In comparison, this age group accounts for about

Table 8.   Special Problems Signalled by the NARD

---

90 case reports of granulocytopenia (1972-77)
        42 (47%) associated with a pyrazole derivative
        20 (22%) associated with metamizol

———

1078 case reports about triazolam 1979
        868 reports on all other drugs in 1979

———

183 case reports of anaphylactic reactions
(oral use, 1980-84)
        121 (66%) associated with glafenine

---

22 % of the total Dutch population. There was a predominance of reports concerning the skin (40%) and the nervous system (28%). The most reported drugs were: amoxicillin and ampicillin (55 reports), valproic acid (21), ketotifen (17), co-trimoxazole (15), salbutamol (14), carbamazepine (14), erythromycin (13), vaccines (12), domperidone (11), and deptropine (11).

The predominance of symptoms of the nervous system suggests that this organ may in childhood be especially susceptible to side effects. Reactions attracting attention were acute extrapyramidal dystonia (metoclopramide, domperidone), hallucinations (oxolamine, deptropine), and agitation (beta-2-sympathomimetics). Blood dyscrasias, erythema multiforme, and hepatic injury - adverse reactions well known to occur in adults - were also reported in children.

Targeted Reporting

When a signal or problem is detected, it can be helpful to request the selective reporting of a specific reaction, in order to try to increase rapidly the knowledge of the nature and the extent of the problem. The attention of health practitioners can, in different ways, be focused on specific subjects. A disadvantage of targeted reporting is, on the other hand, that selective reporting may render a signal less reliable and may blur comparisons between drugs.

"Dear Doctor" letters concerning practolol and triazolam have been sent by the NARD to all doctors and pharmacists. In 1981 the NARD made an inquiry to pulmonologists and allergists with regard to the occurrence of "unexpected sudden death in asthma patients and a possible relationship with the use of medicines."[92] As a result, information was received concerning 27 deaths (and an additional five near-fatal cases). In all but one of these cases the patients had been using beta-2-sympathomimetics (i.e., salbutamol, terbutaline, fenoterol) by inhalation, mostly in overdose. The characteristic sequence of events was: progression of dyspnea, increased use of sympathomimetic inhalations, and subsequently the sudden collapse and death of the patient. Not all patients, however, had had severe dyspnea. Cardiac arrhythmias were reported in eight cases; electrolytes (potassium) were not assessed. The results showed that the occurrence of sudden and unexpected death, in close temporal association with the excessive inhalation of beta-2-sympathomimetics, is a clinical reality, but a causal role of these drugs remained unproven. Presumably different factors may be involved in different patients, e.g., underuse of corticosteroids, overreliance on the inhalation treatment, and the use of toxic doses of sympathomimetics, leading to resistent bronchospasm or cardiac arrhythmia.

An inquiry to nursing homes in the Netherlands provided evidence that an abrupt decrease of blood pressure following the start of antihypertensive treatment in the elderly may cause cerebral ischemia and occasionally stroke.[93]

A small scale inquiry to practitioners involved in the care of elderly patients revealed information on 22 patients with congestive heart failure, possibly induced by the use of nonsteroidal anti-inflammatory drugs.[94]

Advantages and Limitations

The virtues and limitations of Voluntary Reporting are summarized in Table 9. The system has a very broad spectrum, covering all drugs, all patients, and a wide variety of different adverse reactions, is comparatively rapid and cheap, and has been reasonably successful.   An   important   disadvantage,   sometimes   causing   confusion   and misunderstanding, is that the individual case reports are suspicions and not facts. Yet this is a common phenomenon in medicine, since many diagnoses have an aspect of uncertainty. Often this problem can be more or less overcome by studying the reports in interrelationship and comparing the patterns of reported reactions.

Important disadvantages, especially in the Netherlands, are underreporting and the absence of up-to-date consumption figures, which are responsible for the inability of the system to measure the exact frequency of occurrence of reactions and to compare the safety of different drugs. In view of the aims of VR, it may be argued whether this is really a shortcoming. It is now well recognized that the assessment of the frequencies of reactions requires other methods of investigation. VR is especially useful for the study of characteristic reactions with a clear temporal relationship with the drug. Chronic toxicity and delayed effects, on the other hand, often need other methods of assessment, and VR may be of little use when a drug is associated with an increased frequency of a spontaneously occurring disease.

In almost every country there is a large degree of underreporting of adverse reactions to drugs. Even for serious reactions, reporting rates exceeding 30% are rarely achieved.[95] In the Netherlands under-reporting is a comparatively great problem; the annual number of reports is only about 1000 and over a period of three years only about 8% of the doctors submitted at least one adverse reaction report.[96] In the Scandinavian countries, the UK, and also Australia and New Zealand, on the other hand, with a four to five times higher reporting rate, much better figures are achieved. Underreporting is especially a problem because it is very variable and influenced by many different factors; underreporting may differ strongly for different drugs and reactions and changes with time. Experiences in various countries show that, in a country with about 15 million inhabitants, the optimal annual number of case reports is likely to be in the order of magnitude of about 5000 to 10,000. With lower numbers the system is less reliable; with larger numbers the management of the system becomes increasingly expensive but not proportionately more effective. Very large numbers of reports are difficult to handle, may cause delay, and may even blur the picture. Perhaps even more important than the number is the quality of the reports (i.e., the relevance of the reported experiences and the quality of the data in the reports). It takes much energy for a national center to teach a large proportion of the medical practitioners to contribute adequately to its monitoring program, and to achieve a lasting increase in reporting. With only a small staff, such as the NARD's, these goals are difficult to achieve. A good functioning monitoring system is, however, a prerequisite for the safe introduction of new medicines.

USE OF THE DATA

In various ways the data arising from VR can be used for its ultimate aim, the improvement of the safe use of medicines. It is the specific responsibility of a national center such as the NARD that the system is used to its best possible advantage.

Patient Care

The NARD is regularly consulted by practitioners with questions regarding patients with suspected adverse reactions.   These questions usually refer to the possibility, or the likelihood, of a relationship between an adverse event and a drug and to the diagnosis and the further treatment of the patient. When the available literature data are inconclusive (which is not infrequently the case), the file of unpublished experiences may be a useful reference in guiding such problems.

Hypothesis Generation

Experiences in many countries have shown that VR produces a continuous stream of signals concerning suspected adverse drug reactions.   Many of these signals are

Table 9.   Advantages and Limitations of Spontaneous Monitoring

ADVANTAGES	LIMITATIONS

All drugs &
    all patients
 Signal generation &
    serial assessment
 Effective
 Rapid
 Cheap
	Suspicions
	 Underreporting & bias
	 Only characteristic events
	    with temporal relationship
	 - no chronic toxicity
	 - no delayed effects
	 No denominator and no quantification
	 Need for testing of signals

uncertain and too weak for publication, or for for regulatory action, and many suspicions may remain unsubstantiated. Many other hypotheses are serious or interesting enough, however, to deserve further study, for confirmation and clarification, by experimental, pharmacological, or epidemiological investigation. At the NARD the signals are discussed at monthly intervals in a multidisciplinary Advisory Committee, and contact may be made with appropriate research institutions.

When a suspicion is strong and important the immediate notification of the medical and pharmaceutical communities may be needed. In addition to scientific criteria, medical-ethical considerations may be involved in the decision-making. In this respect the support to the NARD of the independent Advisory Committee has proved to be particularly helpful.

Information and Education

It is the NARD's responsibility that adverse reactions are detected and made known as early as possible and at the same time that doubtful data are not disclosed and that false alarms are prevented. Referring to the observations above (see hypothesis generation), a dilemma may arise between the prevention of damage to the patients on the one hand and of damage to the suspected drug on the other. The dissemination of unsubstantiated suspicions is not only likely to disturb the marketing of the drug, but also to damage the repution of the monitoring center and may deter practitioners from further collaboration.

Although with every new adverse reaction the situation is different and a different approach may be needed, with regard to the distribution of information the following observations can be made. In the early phase of a signal, it can be very valuable to exchange experiences with experts in and outside the country, including those working within the pharmaceutical industry, to discuss the possible pharmacological mechanisms and epidemiological aspects. When a suspicion strengthens, often the problem can be solved by adapting the product information (data sheet) and by informing practitioners.

When VR reveals a strong suspicion about a serious adverse reaction, the NARD will consider the need to disseminate information without delay in the professional media, in a special "adverse drug reactions bulletin" or, in the case of an emergency as happened with practolol and triazolam, by mail. These actions not only ensure the availability of relevant information to medical practitioners, but also show the importance of VR and are likely to stimulate participation in the system.

Even when the reported reactions are not new or spectacular, the data obtained by VR has in various respects great educational value. The experiences described in the reports disclose the circumstances in which adverse reactions occur in practice and may yield information which will increase the understanding of adverse drug reactions and improve their prevention. The NARD therefore tries as much as possible to be involved in pre- and postgraduate medical and pharmaceutical training and to intensify the use of the reporting system for educational purposes, in order to serve its ultimate goal: the improvement of the safe use of medicines and the prevention of adverse reactions.

Regulation

Safety is an important element of postmarketing surveillance and drug regulation and, up to the present day, VR plays a key role in this respect. After approval of a new drug, experience steadily increases and new facts are likely to become available, requiring the updating of the approved product information. Many of the new data emanate from anecdotal or systematic reporting and most problems can be solved by adjustment of the data sheet and the inclusion of additional side effects, warnings, contra-indications, and, when needed, narrowing the indications for use. In addition, VR is important in the management of the, fortunately rare, situation when serious problems with adverse reactions require profound restrictions or even the withdrawal of a drug. As has been pointed out before, however, data produced by VR may be an inappropriate basis for the final decision in such instances.

RELATIONS WITH OTHER METHODS

Several other drug monitoring systems exist in the Netherlands, e.g., for skin reactions, malformations, and side effects affecting the eye. A regional system for intensified adverse reaction reporting has already achieved a high response rate. Yet these systems are modified reporting systems. VR is, in the first place, a system for generating signals and hypotheses. Usually many further questions arise, such as the frequency, the mechanisms involved, and possible risk factors. VR should, therefore, be performed in close collaboration with other research activities, including epidemiology, pharmacology, immunology, and pathology. A collaborative study of the NARD on granulocytopenia 10 years ago showed the value of combining data from different sources.[86] The academic community in the Netherlands has in the past been passive with regard to the study of drug safety. Fortunately, recent activities now show a strongly increased interest in pharmacoepidemiology and drug safety. It is to be hoped that these activities will develop, and that the available resources will be used for studies truly contributing to the improvement of the safe and rational use of medicines and of the health of the community.

The further development of pharmacoepidemiology is likely to cause considerable changes in postmarketing surveillance and the place of VR. There is no doubt, however, that VR will continue to play a role, especially with regard to the early detection of rare but important adverse reactions.

SUMMARY

In the Netherlands, as in many other countries, drug regulation and "spontaneous monitoring" or "voluntary reporting" (VR) developed in the early sixties, in the aftermath of the thalidomide tragedy. VR started as an initiative of the medical community in an attempt to create an early warning system to prevent or minimize future drug-induced disasters; the system is now maintained by the governmental Netherlands Centre for Monitoring of Adverse Reactions to Drugs (NARD). In the past decades, while learning by experience and international collaboration, VR has developed into a distinct method, with its principles and procedures, its advantages and limitations. In the meantime the understanding of the complex problems involved in postmarketing surveillance and drug safety studies has improved and additional pharmacoepidemiological methods have been developed.

The most important contribution of VR has been the detection of adverse reactions; in other words it has been demonstrated by experience that VR fulfils, to a certain extent, its original aim. Whereas the strength of VR concerns the unexpected, and rare, but important adverse reactions, it is of little use in the assessment of delayed effects or drug-induced changes in the frequencies of relatively common diseases.

Secondly, VR has been found to be a good starting point for the study of drug-induced diseases. Sometimes the intensive assessment of a single case can already produce valuable information. More importantly, the country-wide reporting system provides a good opportunity for studying relatively large series of cases of rare adverse reactions, enabling the improvement of our knowledge of the clinicopathological features of these disorders. Inherent weaknesses of VR are uncertainty with regard to the causal relationship in most case reports and - large and variable - underreporting, whereas confidentiality and privacy cause some restraints with regard to the use of the data. In the past years the NARD has contributed to publications on about 50 different adverse reactions and interactions.

Additional uses of the data provided by VR are patient care (i.e., by answering questions of health professionals), drug regulation, and (post-graduate) education.

Many signals need further study for confirmation (or refutation), clarification, and quantitative assessment. After a slow start, pharmacoepidemiology is now rapidly developing in the Netherlands and considerable changes in the field of postmarketing surveillance are envisaged. These promising developments are likely to change the place of VR. There is no doubt, however, that a well functioning country-wide VR system will also in the future be a prerequisite for the safe introduction of new medicines.

REFERENCES

1. International Drug Monitoring: The Role of National Centres. World Health Organization Technical Report Series, No. 498, Geneva, 1972.
2. W. H. W. Inman, and E. P. Gill, eds., Monitoring for Drug Safety, Second Edition, 107-118, MTP Press, Lancaster (1986).
3. J. McEwen, and B. Vrhovac, Panel on management of ADR reports in selected national centers, *Drug Information J.* 19:329-44 (1985).
4. J. P. Griffin, and J. C. P. Weber, Voluntary systems of adverse reaction reporting, *in*: "Medicines: Regulation, Research and Risk," J. P. Griffin, P. F. D'Arcy, D. W. G. Harron, eds., Greystone Books Ltd., Antrim (1989).
5. N. Moore, G. Paux, B. Begaud, M. Biour, E. Loupi, F. Boismare, and R. J. Royer, Adverse drug reactions monitoring: doing it the French way, *Lancet.* 2:1056-8 (1985).
6. Drug Monitoring in the Nordic Countries, NLN Publication No 25, Nordic Counsel on Medicines, Box 607, S-75125 Uppsala, Sweden, (1989).
7. M. D. Rawlins, Spontaneous reporting of adverse drug reactions, *Br J Clin Pharmacol.* 26:1-11 (1988).
8. D. M. Davies, History and epidemiology, *in*: "Textbook of adverse drug reactions," D. M. Davies, ed., pp. 3-11, Oxford University Press, Oxford (1985).
9. C. P. H. Van Dijke, and H. Mattie, Bijwerkingen van geneesmiddelen op een afdeling Inwendige Geneeskunde, *Ned Tijdschr Geneeskd.* 130:1889-93 (1986).
10. R. H. B. Meyboom, The Netherlands, *in*: "Monitoring for Drug Safety", W. H. W. Inman, E. P. Gill, eds., Second Editon, pp. 107-118, MTP Press, Lancaster (1986).
11. J. F. Dunne, The World Health Organization, In: "Monitoring for Drug Safety," W. H. W. Inman, E. P. Gill, eds., Second Editon, pp. 165-172, MTP Press, Lancaster (1986).
12. R. H. B. Meyboom, Anafylaxie na het gebruik van geneesmiddelen, *Ned Tijdschr Geneeskd.* 120:926-7 (1976).
13. R. H. B. Meyboom, Merkwaardige verschijnselen tijdens het gebruik van benzydamine (Tantum), *Ned Tijdschr Geneeskd.* 119:1044 (1975).
14. R. H. B. Meyboom, Practolol and sclerosing peritonitis, *Lancet.* 1:334 (1975).
15. R. Van Leeuwen, and R. H. B. Meyboom, Agranulocytosis and aprindine, *Lancet.* 2:1137 (1976).
16. R. Van Leeuwen, Agranulocytose tijdens het gebruik van aprindine, *Ned T Geneeskd.* 120:1549-50 (1976).
17. R. H. B. Meyboom, Psychische stoornissen tijdens het gebruik van triazolam (Halcion), Letter to Dutch physicians and pharmacists, July 16 (1979).
18. H. Dankbaar, and A. H. Mudde, Koorts en leverfunctiestoornissen ten gevolge van nomifensine (Alival), *Ned Tijdschr Geneeskd.* 124:2184 (1980).

19. B. H. C. Stricker, Huidafwijkingen door gebruik van camazepam (Albego), *Ned Tijdschr Geneeskd.* 128:870-2 (1984).
20. B. H. C. Stricker, and C. B. Reith, Ernstige nierfunctiestoornis tijdens gebruik van cimetidine (Tagamet), *Ned Tijdschr Geneeskd* 124:2183-4 (1980).
21. W. H. De Fraiture, F. H. J. Claas, and R. H. B. Meyboom, Bijwerkingen van ticlopidine; klinische waarneming en immunologisch onderzoek, *Ned Tijdschr Geneeskd.* 126:1051-4 (1982).
22. F. H. J. Claas, W. H. De Fraiture, and R. H. B. Meyboom, Thrombopénie causée par des anticorps induits par la ticlopidine, *Nouv Rev Fr Hematol.* 26:323-4 (1984).
23. C. P. H. Van Dijke, Hepatitis tijdens het gebruik van ketoconazol (Nizoral), *Ned Tijdschr Geneeskd.* 127:339-41 (1983).
24. C. P. H. Van Dijke, F. R. Veerman, and H. C. Haverkamp, Anaphylactic reactions to ketoconazole, *Brit Med J.* 287:1673 (1983).
25. B. H. C. Stricker, Slokdarmbeschadiging door pinaveriumbromide, *Ned Tijdschr Geneeskd* 127:603-4 (1983).
26. B. H. C. Stricker, J. N. M. Barendrecht, and F. H. J. Claas, Thrombocytopenia and leucopenia with mianserin-dependent antibodies, *Br J Clin Pharac.* 19:102-4 (1985).
27. M. Van Wijhe, B. H. C. Stricker, and V. S. Reijger, Prolonged apnoea with ketamine, *Brit J Anaesth.* 58:573-4 (1986).
28. J. McEwen, R. H. B. Meyboom, Testicular pain caused by mazindol, *Brit Med J.* 287:1763-4 (1983).
29. R. H. B. Meyboom, More on transderm scop patches, *New Engl J Med.* 311:1377 (1984).
30. B. H. C. Stricker, R. H. B. Meyboom, P. A. Bleeker, Van Wieringen, Blood disorders associated with pirenzepine, *Brit Med J* 293:1074 (1986).
31. W. W. De Herder, P. Schröder, A. Purnode, A. C. M. Van Vliet, B. H. C. Stricker, Pirprofen-associated hepatic injury, *J Hepatol.* 4:127-32 (1987).
32. Hoest, een bijwerking van captopril en enalapril, Bulletin Bijwerkingen Geneesmiddelen, Nr 2, p11-12, June 1986, Ministry of Welfare, Public Health and Culture, Rijswijk, Netherlands.
33. H. M. Markusse, and R. H. B. Meyboom, Gynaecomastia associated with captopril, *Brit Med J.* 296:1262 (1988).
34. B. H. C. Stricker, C. P. H. Van Dijke, A. J. Isaacs, and M. Lindquist, Skin reactions to terfenadine, *Brit Med J.* 293:536 (1986).
35. R. H. B. Meyboom, M. D. Ferrari, and B. P. Dieleman, Parkinsonism, tardive dyskinesia, akathisia, and depression induced by flunarizine, *Lancet.* 2:292 (1986).
36. Overgevoeligheidsreacties op mebendazol, Bulletin Bijwerkingen Geneesmiddelen, Nr 3, p 18-20, June 1987, Ministry of Welfare, Public Health and Culture, Rijswijk, Netherlands.
37. B. H. C. Stricker, H. S. F. Heijermans, H. Braat, and J. Norg, Fever induced by labetolol, *J Am Med Ass.* 256:619-20 (1986).
38. S. Slegers-Karsmakers, B. H. C. Stricker, Anaphylactic reaction to isoflurane. *Anaesthesia.* 43:506-20 (1988).
39. B. H. C. Stricker, and C. Biriell, Skin reactions and fever with indapamide, *Brit Med J.* 295:1313-4 (1987).
40. J. W. G. Van den Broek, B. L. M. Buennemeyer, B. H. C. Stricker, Cholestatische hepatitis door de combinatie amoxicilline en clavulaanzuur (Augmentin), *Ned Tijdschr Geneeskd.* 132:1495-7 (1988).
41. B. H. C. Stricker, G. Slagboom, R. Demaeseneer, V. Slootmaekers, I. Thijs, and S. Olsson, Anaphylactic reactions to cinoxacin, *Brit Med J.* 297:1434-5 (1988).
42. J. I. Roodnat, M. H. Christiaans, W. M. Nugteren-Huying, J. G. Van der Schroeff, P. Van der Zouwen, B. H. C. Stricker, J. J. Weening, and P. C. Chang, Akute Niereninsuffizienz bei der Behandlung der Psoriasis mit Fumarsäure-Estern, *Schweiz Med Wschr.* 119:826-30 (1989).
43. H. Kuiper, R. H. B. Meyboom, and A. Jansen, Voorbijgaande cholelithiasis bij gebruik van ceftriaxon, *Ned Tijdschr Geneeskd.* 132:1857-8 (1988).
44. R. H. B. Meyboom, H. Kuiper, and A. Jansen, Ceftriaxone and reversible cholelithiasis, *Brit Med J* 297:858 (1988).

45.   R. H. B. Meyboom, and N. De Graaf-Breederveld, Budesonide and psychic side effects, *Ann Intern Med.* 109:683 (1988).
46.   W. Hart, and B. H. C. Stricker, Flutamide and hepatitis, *Ann Intern Med.* 110:943-4 (1989).
47.   R. H. B. Meyboom, K. Bonsema, and P. M. Huisman-Klein Haneveld, Kan naproxen de menstruatie verstoren?, *Ned Tijdschr Geneekjd.* 133:1326-7 (1989).
48.   K. Hoogslag, Interactie tussen Prolixan 300 en anticoagulantia, *Ned Tijdschr Geneeskd.* 117:1103 (1973).
49.   A. W. Broekmans, and R. H. B. Meyboom RHB. Potentiëring van het cumarine-effect door amiodaron (Cordarone), *Ned Tijdchr Geneeskd.* 126:1415-7 (1982).
50.   B. H. C. Stricker, J. L. Delhez, Interaction between flurbiprofen and coumarins, *Brit Med J* 285:812 (1982).
51.   R. H. B. Meyboom, Beinvloeding van antistolling door vermageringsproducten, *Tromnibus.* 10(1):3 (1982).
52.   R. H. B. Meyboom, Kunnen geneesmiddelen de betrouwbaarheid van 'de pil' beinvloeden?, *Ned Tijdschr Geneeskd.* 118:1767 (1974).
53.   C. P. H. Van Dijke, J. P. C. Weber, Interaction between oral contraceptives and griseofulvin, *Brit Med J.* 288:1125-6 (1984).
54.   R. H. B. Meyboom, B. W. Pater, Overgevoeligheid voor alcoholische dranken tijdens behandeling met ketoconazol, *Ned Tijdschr Geneeskd.* 133:1463-4 (1989).
55.   G. H. Weenink, C. A. Van Dijk-Wierda, R. H. B. Meyboom, J. G. Koppe, C. R. Staalman, and P. E. Treffers, Teratogeen effect van coumarine-derivaten, *Ned Tijdschr Geneeskd.* 125:702-6 (1981).
56.   D. Lindhout, and H. Meinardi, Gebruik van valproïnezuur gedurende de zwangerschap: een indicatie voor prenataal onderzoek op spina bifida, *Ned Tijdschr Geneesk.* 128:2438-40 (1984).
57.   R. H. B. Meyboom, Icterus door phenprocoumon, *Tromnibus.* 4(1):4 (1976).
58.   R. H. B. Meyboom, Slokdarmbeschadiging door doxycycline en tetracycline, *Ned Tijdschr Geneeskd.* 121:1770 (1977).
59.   B. H. C. Stricker, and R. H. B. Meyboom, Hepatitis bij gebruik van glafenine, *Pharm Weekbld.* 114:405 (1979).
60.   G. Boëtius, A. Stuurman, and J. Bol, Onvruchtbaarheid van de man tijdens behandeling met salazosulfapyridine, *Ned Tijdschr Geneeskd.* 124:1835-6 (1980).
61.   R. H. B. Meyboom, Thrombocytopenia induced by nalidixic acid, *Brit Med J.* 289:962 (1984).
62.   Fotodermatitis door azapropazon (Prolixan), Bulletin Bijwerkingen Geneesmiddelen, Nr 1, p 9-10, July 1985, Ministry of Welfare, Public Health and Culture, Rijswijk, Netherlands.
63.   S. Olsson, C. Biriell, and G. Boman, Photosensitivity during treatment with azapropazone, *Brit Med J.* 291:939 (1985).
64.   B. H. C. Stricker, and T. T. Oei, Agranulocytosis caused by spironolactone, *Brit Med J.* 289:731 (1984).
65.   Hallucinaties door oxolamine, Bulletin Bijwerkingen Geneesmiddelen, Nr 2, p11-12, June 1986, Ministry of Welfare, Public Health and Culture, Rijswijk, Netherlands.
66.   J. McEwen, R. H. B. Meyboom, and I. Thijs, Hallucinations in children caused by oxolamine citrate, *Med J Austr.* 150:449-52 (1989).
67.   R. H. B. Meyboom, A. Van Gent, D. Zinkstok, Nitrofurantoin-induced parotitis, *Brit Med J.* 285:1049 (1982).
68.   B. H. C. Stricker, Leverbeschadiging door valproïnezuur, *Ned Tijdschr Geneeskd.* 126:2111 (1982).
69.   B. H. C. Stricker, R. H. B. Meyboom, and M. Lindquist, Acute hypersensitivity reactions to paracetamol, *Brit Med J.* 291:938-9 (1985).
70.   L. A. Feiner, B. R. Younge, F. J. Kazmier, B. H. C. Stricker, F. T. Fraunfelder, Optic neuropathy and amiodarone therapy, *Mayo Clin Proc.* 62:702-17 (1987).
71.   R. H. B. Meyboom, D. J. Martin, Beïnvloeding van de lichaamstemperatuur door orale anticonceptiva, *Huisarts Wet.* 33:488-90 (1990).
72.   Ernstige plaatselijke reacties op fenylbutazoninjecties, Bulletin Bijwerkingen Geneesmiddelen, Nr 1, p 7-8, July 1985, Ministry of Welfare, Public Health and Culture, Rijswijk, Netherlands.

73. H. Van der Heide, M. A. Ten Haaft, and B. H. C. Stricker, Pancreatitis caused by methyldopa, *Brit Med J.* 282:1930 (1981).

74. R. H. B. Meyboom, and W. A. R. Huijbers, Acute extrapiramidale bewegingsstoornissen bij jonge kinderen en bij volwassenen tijdens het gebruik van domperion, *Ned Tijdschr Geneeskd.* 132:1981-3 (1988).

75. Flebitis door ergotamine, Bulletin Bijwerkingen Geneesmiddelen, Nr 23 p16-17, June 1987, Ministry of Welfare, Public Health and Culture, Rijswijk, Netherlands.

76. Adverse Drug Reactions Advisory Committee, Australian Adverse Drug Reactions Bulletin, June 1988.

77. W. W. Fibbe, F. H. J. Claas, W. Van der Star-Dijkstra, M. R. Schaafsma, R. H. B. Meyboom, and J. H. F. Falkenburg, Agranulocytosis induced by propylthiouracil: evidence of a drug dependent antibody reacting with granulocytes, monocytes and haematopoietic progenitor cells, *Brit J Haematol.* 64:363-73 (1986).

78. E. A. J. M. Schoenmakers, W. J. Riedel, J. J. De Gier, C. P. H. Van Dijke, G. H. Beuman, J. F. O'Hanlon, Het effect van terfenadine op de rijvaardigheid van geselecteerde patienten, Institute for Drugs, Safety and Behaviour, Beeldsnijdersdreef 85, 6216 EA Maastricht, Netherlands.

79. C. P. H. Van Dijke, R. J. Heydendael, M. J. De Kleine, Methimazole, carbimazole, and congenital skin defects, *Ann Intern Med.* 106:60-1 (1987).

80. B. H. C. Stricker, A. P. R. Blok, M. Sinaasappel, J. H. P. Wilson, Het syndroom van Reye in Nederland: verslag van een enquête over de periode 1981-1984, *Ned Tijdschr Geneeskd.* 132:2018-22 (1988).

81. C. M. P. W. Mandigers, F. P. Kroon, R. H. B. Meyboom, Metronidazole is probably safe in patients with G6PD deficiency, Submitted for publication (1990).

82. B. H. C. Stricker, A. P. R. Blok, F. B. Bronkhorst, Glafenine-associated hepatic injury, *Liver* 6:63-72 (1986).

83. B. H. C. Stricker, A. P. R. Blok, F. H. J. Claas, G. E. Van Parijs, V. J. Desmet, Hepatic injury associated with the use of nitrofurans: a clinicopathological study of 52 reported cases, *Hepatology.* 8:559-606 (1988).

84. B. H. C. Stricker, A. P. R. Blok, F. B. Bronkhorst, G. E. Van Parys, V. J. Desmet, Ketoconazole-associated hepatic injury, *J Hepatol.* 3:399-406 (1986).

85. J. H. Lewis, H. J. Zimmerman, G. D. Benson, and K. G. Ishak, Hepatic injury associated with ketoconazole therapy, *Gastroenterology.* 86:503-13 (1984).

86. G. Lake-Bakaar, P. J. Scheuer, and S. Sherlock, Hepatic reactions associated with ketoconazole in the United Kingdom, *Brit Med J.* 294:419-22 (1987).

87. A. Salama, and C. Mueller-Eckhardt, The role of metabolite-specific antibodies in nominfensine-dependent immune hemolytic anemia, *New Engl J Med.* 313:469-74 (1985).

88. F. E. Zwaan, and R. H. B. Meyboom, Causes and consequences of bone marrow insufficiency in man, *Neth J Med* 22:99-104 (1979).

89. R. H. B. Meyboom, De 'Halcion-affaire' in 1979, een loos alarm?, *Ned Tijdschr Geneeskd.* 133:2185-2190 (1989).

90. Acute overgevoeligheidsreacties door geneesmiddelen, Bulletin Bijwerkingen Geneesmiddelen, Nr 3, p 1-11, July 1987, Ministry of Welfare, Public Health and Culture, Rijswijk, Netherlands.

91. R. H. B. Meyboom, Adverse reactions to drugs in children, experiences with "spontaneous motoring" in the Netherlands, *Bratislavské lekársky listy.* (1990) in press.

92. R. H. B. Meyboom, Onverwachte plotseling sterfte van astmapatiënten; resultaten van een enquete, *Ned Tijdschr Geneeskd.* 128457-8 (1984).

93. P. A. F. Jansen, B. P. N. Schulte, R. H. B. Meyboom, and F.W.J. Gribnau, Antihypertensive treatment as a possible cause of stroke in the elderly, *Age and Ageing* 15:129-38 (1986).

94. F. A. Van den Ouweland, F. W. H. Gribnau, and R. H. B. Meyboom, Congestive heart failure as a side effect of nonsteroidal anti-inflammatory drugs in the elderly, *Age and Ageing.* 17:8-16 (1988).

95. J. M. Leiper, and D. H. Lawson, Why do doctors not report adverse drug reactions?, *Neth J Med* 28:546-50 (1985).

96. R. H. B. Meyboom, Het melden van bijwerkingen van geneesmiddelen in Nederland, *Ned Tijdschr Geneeskd.* 130:1879-83 (1986).

PHARMACOVIGILANCE IN FRANCE: A DECENTRALIZED APPROACH

Bernard Begaud, M.D.

Centre de Pharmacovigilance
Hôpital Carreire-Pellegrin
Bordeaux, France

SHORT HISTORY AND STRUCTURE

A decentralized pharmacosurveillance system has been set up in France since 1974.   During the first years (1974 - 1976) reference centers (Centres de Pharmacovigilance) were created in five departments of pharmacology. The role of these centers was to: 1) answer inquiries about drug safety from practitioners, and 2) collect the cases of adverse drug reactions (ADRs) occurring in the area. These centers applied the same principle: a good information service is the best way of getting new information. The number of these "Centres de Pharmacovigilance" increased each year until 1982, date of the official recognition of pharmacovigilance in France by the Decree of July 30th, 1982.

This four page official text (in Journal Officiel de la République Française) summarizes the flow chart and the role of the French Pharmacovigilance as composed of 3 structures:

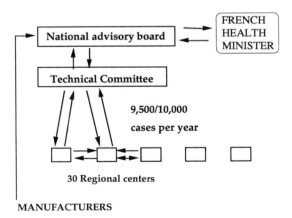

Figure 1.   Structure of French Pharmacovigilance System.

The 30 Regional Centers (Centres Régionaux de Pharmacovigilance)

The geographical distribution of the regional centers (one center in each district capital) maintains an optimal link between the surveillance system and the prescribers. Each center is organized under supervision of a director appointed by the government. The centers have to:

1) collect and assess the ADR cases occurring in their reference area (including public and private practices)
2) answer inquiries (concerning ADRs, drug toxicity, interactions, drugs in pregnancy, etc.) from prescribers, pharmacists, nurses, etc.
3) carry out specific epidemiologic studies in the reference area
4) contribute to methodological research in the field of pharmacosurveillance and ADR diagnosis.

The names of the regional directors and addresses and telephone numbers of the centers are published each year in the French Drug Formulary (Dictionnaire VIDAL des médicaments).

The Technical Committee (Comité Technique de Pharmacovigilance)

The Technical Committee is the bimonthly one day meeting of the 30 regional directors, at the French Health Ministry. The Committee is presided over by one of the 30 directors, chosen for three years by the French Health Minister. The Committee coordinates the work of the 30 regional centers, analyzes the case reports of the previous two month period, discusses the opportunities and methodology of surveys focused on a given drug-event association, and circulates foreign information about drug safety.

The National Advisory Board on Pharmacovigilance (Commission Nationale de Pharmacovigilance)

The National Advisory Board is composed of 27 members and 27 substitutes appointed by the Health Minister, as follows: 10 experts in pharmacology and/or toxicology, 11 physicians (including, at least, three general practitioners), three hospital pharmacists, one chemist, one representative for consumers and one representative for the pharmaceutical industry. The board meets six times per year, and more if necessary; it is presided over by the same person as the National Committee. The Board's main role is to advise the Minister about administrative decisions concerning drug safety: whether to add a warning in the reference books and/or the package insert, to restrict the indications of an approved drug, and to maintain or to withdraw a drug from the market. With the exception of emergency problems, the Board's decisions are based on inquiries prepared by the Technical Committee with the help of the manufacturer concerned.

The Decree of May 24th, 1984 completed the French pharmacovigilance organization by making the reporting of ADR cases mandatory. Prescribers have to report immediately to their regional center all the cases of unexpected adverse drug reactions they observe with drugs they have prescribed (it is not mandatory to report an ADR related to a drug prescribed by another physician). In addition, each year manufacturers have to send to the National Board all the reports they receive involving drugs they market in France (twice a year for recently marketed drugs).

DISTINCTIVE CHARACTERISTICS

Even if the basic scheme is the same as in other developed countries (to centralize reports for decision making), the system set up in France over the past 16 years greatly differs from those conducted by the main regulatory agencies elsewhere (CSM, FDA, BGA, etc.).

First, the regulatory agency is centralized for administrative and political decisions (National Board, Technical Committee), but decentralized for routine activities, especially for drug surveillance. This facilitates interface with prescribers: each center deals with a population ranging from 1.5 to 3 million inhabitants and about 5,000 physicians.

Second, the regional centers are both drug information centers and surveillance units. This is certainly the best way of picking up new ADRs and focusing on relevant information. Prescribers call the center when they observe a "strange" reaction, previously unknown by them and not described in reference books (about 50 % of reports received were initially questions concerning a possible drug reaction). This explains how the system filters for the more interesting ADRs occurring and avoids too great a level of background noise (intensive reporting of perfectly known reactions) due to the mandatory character of reporting: 29.71% of reactions reported during 1989 were not previously described in Meyler's Side Effects of Drugs, Martindale, and Dictionnaire Vidal.

Third, the majority of reports come directly from prescribers: 97.5 % for 1989; only 2 % come from other health professionals and less than 0.2 % from consumers (data from the Bordeaux Center). This medicalization guarantees the better clinical quality of the reports and allows a follow up of the cases.

Fourth, each report is assessed before recording. In 1978, a standardized method for assessing the causal relationship between drug and event was published. In 1984, this method was updated and its use made mandatory for centers and manufacturers for all case reports. The principle is to assess the relationship to *each drug taken by the patient* by scoring 7 criteria (3 criteria for chronology: challenge, dechallenge and rechallenge; 4 criteria for clinical conditions). A combination table provides a global score from 0 (excluded) to 4 (highly probable). The mandatory use of this method has three main advantages:

1) it reduces the background noise by rejection of very improbable or spurious cases;
2) by using the same case analysis, it facilitates exchanges between centers and manufacturers;
3) the method leads the expert to complete information for each criterion; this greatly increases the quality of reports.

Over the last 5 years, the distribution of scores for 65,386 recorded reactions were as follows:

O = NOT RELATED: 993 (1.5 %) only for concomitant drugs
1 = DOUBTFUL : 38,962 (59.6 %)
2 = POSSIBLE : 17,401 (26.6 %)
3 = PROBABLE : 7,366 (11.3 %)
4 = HIGHLY PROBABLE : 663 (1 %)

The overrepresentation of causal relationships assessed as DOUBTFUL reflects the severity of the method and the high proportion of severe reactions (deaths or sequelae) for which it is difficult to score a dechallenge.

ACTIVITY

Each center receives an annual governmental grant correlated to the importance of its activity: number of answers to inquiries, number of cases recorded in the data bank, number of publications, and contributions to scientific progress.

Centers are located in departments of pharmacology or toxicology. The number of people working in a center greatly varies from one center to another (from 2 to 12). Including full time and part time salaries, the total number of people working in the 30 centers ranges from 120 to 150 M.D.'s and pharmacists (not including secretaries and other people).

Each center has one or several specific telephone lines devoted to prescribers' calls. The cases are assessed by the center's medical staff and recorded in a central database, which is connected to the 30 centers and the French Health Ministry. The pharmacovigilance database only includes reports from regional centers; the reports

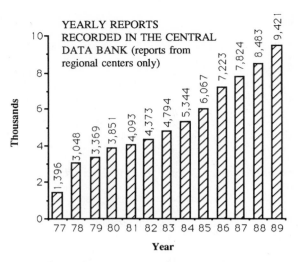

Figure 2.   Annual Reports of ADRs.

transmitted by manufacturers are analyzed separately by the National Board.   The number of reports validated and recorded in 1989 was 9,421. The terminals are micro-computers, allowing local analysis of data extracted from the database. The computer files include at least 33 items with an imputability and a bibliographical score.

Comparisons to the performance of other national systems are very misleading if we forget that

1)   French statistics are only based on reports to the centers and do not consider reports coming through manufacturers (domestic or foreign) or published cases, as is done by the FDA, and

2)   invalid cases or cases with insufficient information are not computerized.

Despite that, the reporting rate in France is roughly comparable to that in the United States, United Kingdom, and Germany (15 to 20 reports per 100,000 inhabitants).

THE USE OF VITAL AND MORBIDITY STATISTICS FOR THE DETECTION

OF ADVERSE DRUG REACTIONS AND FOR MONITORING OF DRUG SAFETY

Paul D. Stolley, M.D., M.P.H.

Department of Epidemiology and Preventive Medicine
University of Maryland School of Medicine
Baltimore, Maryland 21201

In medical practice the clinician is primarily interested in the prevention, diagnosis, and treatment of disease in the individual patient. While the epidemiologist is also interested in disease prevention, diagnosis, and treatment, he focuses on the distribution and determinants of disease in populations and communities rather than on the individual patient. It is this broader perspective that has sometimes enabled epidemiologists to uncover adverse drug reactions, revealed by variations in the geographic, seasonal, or age distribution patterns of certain diseases and, particularly, by changes in the secular trends of disease as revealed by scrutiny of vital statistics and morbidity rates.

Examples of the use of vital statistics in drug epidemiology are not numerous, but several will be described to illustrate the utility and practical applications of this approach.

EPIDEMIC OF DEATHS AMONG ASTHMATIC CHILDREN ATTRIBUTED TO OVERUSE OF POTENT NEBULIZERS

The death rates for asthma remained remarkably stable for an entire century prior to 1960 in the United Kingdom. These rates were low, the crude death rate hovering around 0.5 deaths per 100,000 persons. In 1961, the death rates began to rise rapidly, especially the age-specific rates for ages 5-34 years. After 1967, the death rates for asthma began to decline and in the 1970s almost approached the pre-epidemic levels. A remarkably similar pattern was noted in Scotland, Australia, and Ireland.[1]

After the epidemic was noted by routine perusal of vital statistics records collected by the Office of the Registrar General for England and Wales, specific epidemiologic investigations were initiated to uncover the cause of this sudden increase in mortality.

It was soon established that changes in disease nomenclature and the coding of death certificates could not account for the increasing rates. An investigation of the circumstances surrounding the deaths of asthmatic children in and around London suggested that use and/or abuse of isoproterenol-containing nebulizers was implicated.[2] Additional studies correlating the introduction and increasing sales of this medication with the increasing death rates gave additional support to this hypothesis. Because certain countries such as the United States of America and Canada sold large amounts of these nebulizers and yet were spared the epidemic, these exceptions tended to erode acceptance of the "nebulizer hypothesis" as the most likely explanation for the epidemic of asthma deaths. However, these exceptions were explained by an international comparative study of asthma death rates and nebulizer sales.[1] This report demonstrated

Drug Epidemiology and Post-Marketing Surveillance, Edited by B.L. Strom
and G. Velo, Plenum Press, New York, 1992

that sales of a superpotent nebulizer five times stronger than the usual formulation were strongly associated with both the presence and extent of the epidemic. This very potent formulation was not licensed or marketed in the U.S.A. and Canada, countries which were spared the epidemic even though they consumed large amounts of the usual (lower) strength nebulizer formulations.[3]

Several mechanisms have been postulated to explain in physiological terms the deaths apparently related to the use of these adrenergic medications. While there is no general consensus, the most likely explanation is that the potent nebulizers delivered doses large enough to cause fatal tachycardias in children already compromised by hypoxemia and often primed with other cardiotonic drugs such as theophylline.[4]

In any event, the epidemic began to wane as sales of the nebulizers declined because of warnings about their hazards and substitution by newer medications with more selective adrenergic effects less liable to induce tachycardias.[3]

This account of the epidemic of asthma deaths illustrates the value of vital statistics for the recognition of epidemics and the use of drug sales and consumption data in the elucidation of the probable cause of the epidemic.

STUDIES OF MORTALITY TRENDS FOR THROMBOEMBOLISM, PULMONARY EMBOLISM, AND MYOCARDIAL INFARCTION AS CORRELATED WITH ORAL CONTRACEPTIVE USE

After the first case reports had appeared casting suspicion on the oral contraceptives as possibly increasing the risk of deep vein thrombosis and consequent pulmonary embolism, several case-control (retrospective) investigations were launched. Prior to undertaking such a case-control study in the U.S.A., Sartwell and Anello[5] first examined death rates attributable to thromboembolism and pulmonary embolism from 1960-66 to determine if trends in these rates were consistent with the hypothesis that OCs increased the risk of developing (and dying from) these diseases.

Their analysis showed an increase in death rates due to venous thromboembolism and pulmonary embolism beginning shortly after the introduction of the oral contraceptives (about 1960-61) in women at risk, i.e., in the child-bearing age groups. Older women and men did not show this pattern. These findings were consistent with the hypothesis of increased risk due to use of the OCs and encouraged Sartwell and his colleagues to proceed with their case-control investigation which showed a fourfold increased risk of pulmonary embolism in association with antifertility agents.[5]

North American, English, and Swedish investigators collaborated on a study of death due to pulmonary embolism where they compared the estrogen dose of the pills used by the deceased with the "expected" use as estimated from sales data. Finding an excess use of high estrogen dosage forms, they concluded that it was probably this component (rather than the progestin) which increased the risk of thrombotic disease, and recommended a switch to the low-dose estrogen formulation OCs.[6] Some years later, the efficacy of this public health measure was evaluated by Sartwell and Stolley[7] who examined U.S.A. death statistics and showed a falloff in death rates for pulmonary embolism in women following the switch to the lower-dose OCs.

Other studies of death rates for stroke and myocardial infarction as related to OC usage patterns have shown a similar pattern, but less consistently and less conclusively than is the case for pulmonary embolism.[8]

This example illustrates how vital statistics and drug sales data can be used to examine the consistency of such information with hypotheses of drug-induced disease causation. Specific analytic studies, both case-control and cohort investigations, were required to confirm these hypotheses, but the vital statistics data gave some support to these explanations and were important ancillary evidence. They also helped evaluate the effect of a specific public health measure, i.e., the switch to oral contraceptives with a lower dose of estrogen.

SUBACUTE MYELO-OPTIC NEUROPATHY (SMON)

This unusual neurologic disease was unexplained until Japanese investigators linked its occurrence to ingestion of the halogenated hydroxyquinoline drugs commonly used to treat and prevent nonspecific gastroenteritis. This "new" disease had a seasonal pattern in Japan and so an infectious etiology was suspected at first.[9]   Further epidemiologic investigation showed the victims of the disease frequently gave a history of prior ingestion of large doses of the hydroxyquinolines, and the seasonal incidence pattern was also explained by the seasonal pattern of the disease, gastroenteritis, for which the drug is used. Disease incidence and sales of the drug correlated closely, and when the drug was eventually banned from use by the Japanese government, the disease virtually disappeared as drug use ceased, falling from over fifty reported cases to less than five in two months.[10]

Subsequently, animal experiments conclusively linked the drug to the disease, as it could be reliably reproduced in a dog "model".

This example illustrates the occasional use of morbidity statistics in an "experiment of prevention"; the drug is removed from distribution and use and the disease may disappear.

METHYLDOPA AND BILIARY DUCT CARCINOMA

A Swedish report implicated the antihypertensive drug methyldopa as a possible cause of cancer of the biliary ducts.[11] This investigation compared the frequency of drug use in cases of this tumor to use frequency that would have been "expected" based on national sales records.

In an attempt to seek support for this hypothesis, Strom et al.[12] examined secular trends for this tumor assembled from a number of tumor registries around the world. These incidence rates over time were then compared to methyldopa sales in the corresponding regions. The hypothesis of drug causation in regard to the etiology of this cancer received no support from this type of analysis. Although drug sales had grown markedly in some areas over the past two decades, the incidence rates for the tumor tended to remain relatively constant and did not increase, even after taking into account various "lag-times" since drug introduction.

This example shows how vital statistics and disease registries can be used in conjunction with drug sales data to shed light on the plausibility of a hypothesis linking drug use to a disease. Of course, this evidence is weaker than that obtained from appropriately designed and conducted case-control or cohort analytic investigations.

THALIDOMIDE AND PHOCOMELIA

The well-known episode of thalidomide-induced congenital malformations is briefly described here because of the less-known contribution that malformation registries made to the understanding of the epidemic. Ingestion of thalidomide, a mild hypnotic, by pregnant women during their first trimester may lead to the birth of children with absent parts of their limbs, a condition called phocomelia. While the epidemic of phocomelia and its connection with thalidomide was observed by an astute pediatrician,[13] examination of data from malformation registries helped confirm the original observations.

Recording data on the type and frequency of malformations and linking these data with thalidomide sales convincingly showed that both the appearance and disappearance of this unusual anomaly coincided with sales of thalidomide, with the sales preceding the malformations from eight months to a year.[14]

SACCHARIN, CYCLAMATES, AND BLADDER CANCER

Rodent experiments strongly suggested that saccharin, a non-nutritive artificial sweetener, was a bladder carcinogen for certain species. Case-control epidemiologic studies in humans examining this question had been inconclusive, showing discrepant results. Vital statistics and cancer incidence data from tumor registries have been helpful in considering this issue. In the U.S.A., "soda" beverages containing cyclamates and saccharin became very popular in the 1960s and 1970s. Furthermore, persons with diabetes mellitus are thought to consume more non-nutritive artificial sweeteners than nondiabetics. If the artificial sweeteners were important causes of bladder cancer, an increased incidence might be expected some years after their introduction and widespread use; and diabetics might exhibit a higher incidence of this tumor than nondiabetics.

Analysis of bladder cancer incidence rates both in the general population and among diabetics does not show any "artificial sweetener effect." A slow and constant rise in male incidence of bladder cancer is noted, consistent with changes in cigarette smoking habits, cigarette smoking being a known risk factor.[15]

This example shows how examination of disease rates in special populations heavily exposed to the suspected drug or chemical can be a useful adjunct to other investigations.

DIETHYLSTILBESTROL AND ADENOCARCINOMA OF THE VAGINA IN ADOLESCENT GIRLS

Diethylstilbestrol (DES), a synthetic nonsteroidal estrogen, is a potent carcinogen in several animal species. DES had been used in medical practice for three decades and had been added to animal feeds for about fifteen years. Its medical uses have included a variety of gynecologic conditions in which estrogen replacement was deemed necessary as, for example, in the treatment of certain symptoms of menopause. It was used in cattle feed because it brings the animal to slaughter at a higher weight in a shorter period of time and at less cost of feed. There is some argument as to whether the increased weight gain in cattle is due to fat deposition or to increased muscular growth (protein), but the DES is thus ingested by the consumer in small amounts. In January 1973, the Food and Drug Administration (FDA) prohibited the addition of DES to cattle feed after one of the more acrimonious scientific debates of recent years.

But DES had another use in medical practice in the United States in the 1940s and 1950s, and it was this use (whose efficacy to increase fetal salvage in habitual aborters was later disproven, incidentally) that led to the appearance of a minor "epidemic" of vaginal cancer in the daughters 15 to 20 years after the ingestion of DES by their mothers. The practice which developed among obstetricians in the 1940s of administering high doses of DES to the pregnant women, especially during the first trimester, is supported in the literature of that time by a number of favorable reports of an uncontrolled series of patients and a few poorly controlled studies. Finally, at the end of the 1950s, a well-controlled randomized double-blind trial showed no benefit. The popularity of the DES prophylaxis then declined in obstetric practice.

The use of DES in pregnancy in high doses had been particularly advocated by a prestigious group in the Boston area, where it gained fairly wide acceptance; and so it was in this area that the minor "epidemic" was first noted: eight cases of adenocarcinoma of the vagina in women under 20 years of age were treated in a single Boston hospital within a five-year time span, 1966-71. Prior to 1966, not a single case of this type of cancer in that younger age group had ever been treated at this hospital. This clustering of a rare disease in an unusual age group, in time and locale, obviously represented an unusual phenomenon and was investigated by Herbst, Ulfelder, and Poskanzer[16]. A case-control retrospective study showed an association of maternal ingestion of DES with subsequent cancer in the progeny. None of the 32 "control" mothers had taken this drug.

Since this study, an uncontrolled series of over 500 additional cases has been reported to an ad hoc vaginal cancer registry, and about three-quarters have histories of maternal ingestion of DES or one of its congeners.[17] It should be noted that DES is still available and used as a "morning after pill," i.e., a postcoital contraceptive.

The DES-induced vaginal cancer story points up the value of establishing a disease registry when a "new" disease or altered disease pattern is noted. The registry would have been more useful if a "control" or comparison group were simultaneously collected. The comparison group would permit inferences concerning dosage, time given in pregnancy, duration of use, and other measures of risk associated with this drug-induced tumor.[18]

ENDOMETRIAL CANCER AND EXOGENOUS ESTROGENS

Numerous case-control epidemiologic investigations have firmly linked the use of exogenous estrogens to an increased risk of endometrial carcinoma. When this association was first suspected, examination of secular trends for uterine cancer failed to show the increase expected in relation to the increasing sales and use of these estrogens. It was soon realized that failure to see a rise in uterine cancer following the widespread use of estrogens in the 1960s in the U.S.A. was due to improper calculation of incidence and mortality rates. If one calculates age-specific or crude rates of this tumor for women, the denominator for these rates will include women who have undergone hysterectomy and thus are not truly at risk of developing this tumor, no longer having uteri. This incorrect denominator would not have been misleading if hysterectomy were an uncommon procedure--but such is not the situation in the U.S.A. where hysterectomy is a very common procedure in middle-aged women (along with the mounting popularity of estrogen supplements) and became increasingly frequent in the 1960s.

In 1974, for example, the uncorrected incidence rate per 100,000 for cancer of the corpus uteri, in white females of Alameda County, California, was 50/100,000; when the denominator was changed to exclude women who had had hysterectomies, the incidence rate jumped to 72/100,000. The true magnitude of the problem was masked by use of the improper denominator when calculating these rates and the correction reveals a more striking increase following closely the increased use of estrogens over time.[19]

CONCLUSION

It can be seen that a study of the appearance of "new" diseases, changes in the incidence of older or well-described diseases, their geographic distribution, age distribution, and the ongoing rise and fall of diseases may all give clues about drug-related effects. Drug-monitoring systems, the routine collection of vital statistics, and observations by astute clinicians all contribute to the uncovering and understanding of drug-induced disease. Accurate and reliable sources of information about geographic differences in morbidity, mortality, and drug utilization will provide the "intelligence system" needed to help detect unwanted and unanticipated drug reactions. Geographic differences in the marketing or use of such drugs as oral hypoglycemics, anabolic androgens, oral contraceptives, reserpine, and estrogens (as used in menopause) might help us detect possible adverse reactions to these agents, all of which are suspected. Changes in disease incidence or emergence of new syndromes in areas where these drugs are heavily used could be contrasted to areas where they are seldom used. Unfortunately, at present this kind of information is seldom available when needed.

REFERENCES

1.   P. D. Stolley, Asthma mortality: why the United States was spared an epidemic of deaths due to asthma, *Am Rev Resp Dis*. 105:883-890 (1972).
2.   P. Fraser, and R. Doll, Geographic variations in the epidemic of asthma deaths, *Br J Preven Soc Med*. 25:34-36 (1971).
3.   P. D. Stolley, and R. Schinnar, Association between asthma mortality and isoproterenol in aerosols: a review, *Preven Med*. 7:519-538 (1978).
4.   J. M. Collins, D. G. McDevitt, R. G. Shanks, and J. G. Swanton, The cardiotoxicity of isoprenaline during hypoxia, *Br J Pharmacol*. 36:35-45 (1969).
5.   P. E. Sartwell, and C. Anello, Trends in mortality from thromboembolic disorders, Second report on the oral contraceptives by Advisory Committee on Obstetrics and Gynecology, Food and Drug Administration, Government Printing Office, Washington, D.C., Appendix 2B, 37-40 (1969).

6. W. H. Inman, M. P. Vessey, B. Westerholm, and A. Engelund, Thromboembolic disease and the steroidal content of oral contraceptives. A report to the Committee on Safety of drugs, *Br Med J*. 2:203-209 (1970).

7. P. E. Sartwell, P. D. Stolley, J. A. Tonascia, M. S. Tockman, A. H. Rutledge, and D. Wertheimer, Overview: pulmonary embolism mortality in relation to oral contraceptive use, *Preven Med*. 5:15-19 (1976).

8. B. L. Strom, and P. D. Stolley, Vascular and cardiac risks of steroidal contraception, *in*: "Gynecology and Obstetrics," Vol. VI, J. W. Sciarra, ed., Harper & Row, Hagerstown, Maryland (1982).

9. T. Tsubaki, Y. Honma, and M. Hoshi, Epidemiological study related to clioquinol as etiology of SMON, *Jap Med J*. 2448:29-34 (1971).

10. G. P. Oakley, The neurotoxicity of the halogenated hydroxyquinolines: a commentary, *JAMA*. 225:395-397 (1973).

11. G. Broden, and L. Bengtsson, Biliary carcinoma associated with methyldopa therapy, *Acta Chir Scand*. Suppl. 500:7-12 (1980).

12. B. L. Strom, P. L. Hibberd, and P. D. Stolley, Methyldopa and biliary carcinoma: an international study of secular trends, *Clin Pharmacol Therap*. 31:273, (1982).

13. W. G. McBride, Thalidomide and congenital abnormalities, (Letter to the Editor), *Lancet*. 2:1358 (1961).

14. H. Sjostrom, and R. Nilsson, "Thalidomide and the Power of the Drug Companies," Penguin Books, Ltd., Middlesex, England (1972).

15. F. Burbank, and J. F. Fraumeni, Synthetic sweetener consumption and bladder cancer trends in the United States, *Nature*. 227:296-297 (1970).

16. A. L. Herbst, H. Ulfelder, and D. C. Poskanzer, Adenocarcinoma of the vagina: association of maternal stilbestrol therapy with tumor appearances in young women, *N Engl J Med*. 284:878-881 (1971).

17. A. L. Herbst, H. A. Bern, and eds., "Developmental Effects of Diethylstilbestrol (DES) in Pregnancy," Thieme-Stratton, New York (1981).

18. S. Shapiro, and D. Slone, The effects of exogenous female hormones on the fetus, *Epidem Rev*. 1:110-123 (1979).

19. J. L. Lyon, and J. W. Gardner, The rising frequency of hysterectomy: its effects on uterine cancer rates, *Am J Epidemiol*. 105:439-443 (1977).

THE USE OF CASE-CONTROL STUDIES IN PHARMACOEPIDEMIOLOGY

Paul D. Stolley, M.D., M.P.H.

Department of Epidemiology and Preventive Medicine
University of Maryland School of Medicine
Baltimore, Maryland 21201

The case-control method of epidemiologic investigation has proven to be of great use in studies of adverse drug reactions and may even have a small role in the assessment of drug benefit as well. The drug history of persons with a condition suspected of being related to drug exposure is compared to the drug history of a suitable comparison group, called a "control group," and the differences in the proportion exposed are measured.

A typical example of the method in practice is illustrated by the first case-control study investigating the etiology of clear-cell adenocarcinoma of the vagina in young women.[1] Two hypotheses were seriously considered by these investigators: that the cancer might be associated with 1) radiation exposure, or 2) drug exposure. Eight cases were compared to 32 controls, the controls being girls born within a few days of the cases and in the same hospital. Table 1 below shows the results of this study when the history of maternal exposure to diethylstilbestrol (DES) was compared.

In this example, the measure of association, the odds ratio, cannot be calculated, because one of the cells of this four-cell table contains a zero. If a 1.0 is added to each cell, the odds ratio (which approximates the relative risk) is calculated by the formula ad/bc and is 132 in this example. This can be interpreted as indicating that a young woman who was exposed to DES *in utero* is 132 times more likely to develop clear-cell adenocarcinoma than a young woman who has not undergone this exposure. The odds ratio measures the odds of the disease in the exposed (drug-takers) relative to the odds of the disease in the non-exposed (those whose mothers did not take the drug).

The case-control method has proven remarkably useful and reliable in studies of the adverse effects and unexpected benefits of the oral contraceptives,[2] post-menopausal estrogen use,[3] the relation of aspirin to Reye's syndrome,[4] relation of toxic shock syndrome to tampon use[5] and very recently, the association of the eosinophilia-myalgia syndrome to ingestion of the food supplement L-tryptophan.[6]

However, the case-control method can present difficulties for the investigator, such as: (1) How reliably can the history of drug use be obtained? (2) What is the most suitable comparison group? (3) What are the sources of bias and can this bias be minimized? (4) What are the potential confounders and can they be controlled? (5) How does one interpret small odds ratios surrounded by wide confidence intervals?

The source of controls for case-control studies can be the same neighborhood or community as the cases, the hospital, or randomly selected subjects from the community using electoral roles or similar listings of residents (or even random digit-dialling techniques).

A confounding variable or a potential confounder is handled in the analysis by multivariate statistical adjustment techniques or stratification. Confounding can be handled in the design by use of matching or exclusion.[7] Current advice is to make

Table 1.   The Use of DES by the Mother While Pregnant and Carrying the Female Subject

	Cases of Vaginal Cancer	Controls
DES Used	7 (a)	0 (b)
DES Not Used	1 (c)	32 (d)
Total:	8	32

$$\text{Odds Ratio} = \frac{ad}{bc}$$

Adapted from reference 1.

If 1.0 is added to each cell, then

$$\text{OR} = \frac{ad}{bc} = \frac{8 \times 33}{2 \times 1} = \frac{264}{2} = 132$$

minimal use of matching in the design because matching can lead to a loss of analytical options and an increase in logistical difficulty in implementing the study.

Bias can be minimized in case-control research by training interviewers to obtain histories of drug use in an even-handed manner from both cases and controls and by keeping subjects and interviewers ignorant of the hypothesis of interest; but the latter advice is often impractical.

Confounding by "indication" is the great bug-bear of drug-reaction epidemiological research and various strategies have been developed to examine it. For example, in studies of Reye's syndrome and salicylate use, matching by severity of prodromal illness or height of fever has been used as well as multi-variate analysis controlling for these variables.[4]

In addition to *ad hoc* studies examining drug/disease etiological hypotheses, continuing case-control surveillance systems have been inaugurated and proven productive in both the testing and generation of hypotheses. Automated data bases have been useful in locating both cases of rare diseases and suitable controls and case-control studies can be performed within the context of large cohorts to reduce the cost of obtaining relevant information on all cohort members (were this technique not utilized).[8]

Once drug/disease associations are uncovered, various criteria are applied to the finding to judge whether or not the association is likely to be of a causal nature. These criteria include the magnitude of the association or relative risk, the consistency of the finding, the biological plausibility of the association, and the temporal relationship of the disease to drug administration.[9]

Small relative risks associating drugs to disease must be interpreted with great caution, most especially if the confidence intervals surrounding these risks are wide. It is in these situations that investigators have been most often misled and drugs have been implicated as the cause of disease and later this has been refuted. The relationship of coffee to pancreatic cancer and reserpine to breast cancer are examples of this over-interpretation of marginal findings.[10,11]

Sample size requirements for case-control studies make this design ideally suited for the study of diseases of low incidence. This is because the incidence of the disease of interest does not figure into the calculation of study size, in contrast to the cohort design. It is rather the prevalence of exposure or use of the suspect drug in the control population that enters into the calculation of study size.[12] If a drug is very rarely used, the study will have to be larger than if the drug is commonly used. Ubiquitous drug use, close to 100 percent, as may be seen for salicylates in some countries, will also mandate a large study.

The case-control method has had a distinguished history in the study of adverse drug reactions. For over three decades, it has evolved to such an extent that it is now recognized as one of the most useful research methods available to investigators. It is instructive to read the comments on the very first case-control studies in the field of drug epidemiology, those studies showing an association between oral contraceptives and thromboembolic disease and uterine cancer and estrogen supplementation. Many of the critics were clearly confused by the method and had only a faint understanding of the nature of confounding and the ways in which it could be controlled. Statisticians trained only in the experimental method and emphasizing the importance of randomization were especially skeptical. Indeed, even the famous Sir Ronald Fisher had great difficulty grappling with the method when it was used by Doll and Hill in their landmark investigations of cigarette-smoking and lung cancer.[13] However, in spite of the criticism, the method has been usually applied and much of what we know of adverse drug reactions and un-anticipated benefit of drugs is a direct result of the application of the method. This is the past history--but what of the future?

It is my belief that the case-control method will continue to be used to answer a number of questions that cannot be feasibly approached in any other way. Drug reactions of very low incidence cannot be studied easily using the cohort method, where study size is determined by the incidence of the disease in the control group. Randomized controlled trials are usually not possible when studying toxic effects and these prospective studies also suffer from the need to be unmanageably large (if the disease incidence is low). The problem of drug history recall common to the case-control method may be partially solved by a reliance on drug histories recorded in an automated data base at the time of prescription-filling. The greater understanding of the strengths and limitations of multi-variate analysis may help to better adjust for confounders in the analysis, and experience with biased information sources will lead to better ways of minimizing such biased information collection.

REFERENCES

1. A. L. Herbst, H. Ulfelder, and D. C. Poskanzer, Registry of clear cell carcinoma of genital tract in young women, N Engl J Med 285:407 (1974).
2. Royal College of General Practitioners, Oral Contraceptives and Health, Pitman, New York (1974).
3. H. K. Ziel, and W. D. Finkle, Increased risk of endometrial carcinoma among users of conjugated estrogens, N Engl J Med 293:1167 (1975).
4. E. S. Hurwitz, M. J. Barrett, D. Bregman, and et. al., Public Health Service study on Reye's syndrome and medication, Report of the pilot phase, N Engl J Med 313:849 (1985).
5. R. A. Stallones, A review of the epidemiologic studies of toxic shock syndrome, Ann Intern Med 96:917 (1982).
6. E. A. Belongia, C. W. Hedberg, G. J. Gleich, and et. al., An investigation of the cause of the eosinophilia-myalgia syndrome associated with tryptophan use, N Engl J Med 323:357-366 (1990).
7. J. J. Schlesselman, Case-Control Studies: Design, Conduct, Analysis, Oxford University Press, New York (1982).
8. J. L. Carson, B. L. Strom, L. Morse, S. L. West, K. A. Soper, P. D. Stolley, and J. K. Jones, The relative gastrointestinal toxicity of nonsteroidal anti-inflammatory drugs. Arch Intern Med 147:1054-1059 (1987).
9. A. B. Hill, Principles of Medical Statistics, 1st Ed. Oxford University Press, Oxford (1937).
10. B. MacMahon, S. Yen, and D. Trichopoulos, Coffee and cancer of the pancreas, N Engl J Med 304:630-633 (1981).
11. Boston Collaborative Surveillance Program, Reserpine and breast cancer, Lancet 2:669 (1974).
12. J. J. Schlesselman, Sample size requirements in cohort and case-control studies of disease, Am J Epidemiol 99:381 (1974).
13. R. Doll, and A. Hill, Smoking and carcinoma of the lung, Brit Med J ii:739 (1950).

THE USE OF COHORT STUDIES IN PHARMACOEPIDEMIOLOGY

Terri H. Creagh, M.S., M.S.P.H.

Clinical Manager
AIDS Research Consortium of Atlanta, Inc.
Atlanta, Georgia 30308

DEFINITION AND TYPES OF COHORT STUDIES

In Epidemiology, cohort studies are generally thought of as being prospective, i.e., individuals in a subset of a population are classified according to their exposure to a specific factor and are then followed to determine whether a particular disease or outcome develops. In this sense, the cohort is defined as a group of individuals who share some kind of common exposure within a defined period of time. In pharmacoepidemiology, a cohort study involves a subset of a specific population in which the members share an exposure to a particular drug or type of intervention. They are followed over time with the purpose of comparing them to some unexposed control group or historical cohort to define the incidence of adverse drug events and/or measures of effectiveness of the drug or intervention. Cohort studies are useful to investigate multiple outcomes from a single exposure, e.g., a newly marketed drug.

A pharmacoepidemiologic cohort study can be prospective, retrospective, or ambispective. A prospective cohort study is one which is performed simultaneous with the clinical events under study. Patient outcome is unknown at the time of the study's initiation. The "gold standard" of a prospective pharmacoepidemiologic study is a double-blind, randomized, placebo-controlled clinical trial. Although the clinical trial is often not thought of as being a pharmacoepidemiologic study, it is clearly the ideal way to apply epidemiologic methods to study the effects and uses of drugs in human populations. Randomization should minimize, but may not necessarily eradicate, confounding and other types of bias which are present in studies of any population.

A retrospective study is one which studies exposures and events which occur prior to the initiation of the study. Importantly, in a retrospective cohort study, patients are still recruited into the study on the basis of the presence or absence of exposure. This contrasts with a retrospective case-control study, in which a group of people exhibiting an event which may be drug-related is compared to a suitable control group not having the event with respect to a previous exposure to the drug in question. Both groups must have a clinical disease or condition, as well as other characteristics, which give each group an equal likelihood of exposure to the drug. For instance, among individuals with osteoarthritis, those who also developed peptic ulcers could be compared to those for whom no ulcers had been reported with respect to exposure to a specific nonsteroidal anti-inflammatory agent.

We can illustrate an ambispective cohort study with our multicenter intensive postmarketing surveillance study which follows a group of patients with advanced human immunodeficiency virus (HIV) disease treated with zidovudine (RETROVIR®, AZT).[1] In late 1987, we began identifying every patient ever presenting with a diagnosis of HIV disease in each clinical site; this included patients who had died or had been lost to

Drug Epidemiology and Post-Marketing Surveillance, Edited by B.L. Strom
and G. Velo, Plenum Press, New York, 1992

follow-up. From this population, a subset of all patients ever treated with zidovudine who met protocol criteria was selected. The further requirement that zidovudine therapy must have been initiated between April 15, 1987, and April 14, 1988, defined a final cohort of approximately 1000 patients in 12 clinical sites. In limiting the study to patients whose therapy began within a defined period of time, we could minimize the effects of secular trends in therapy of HIV disease. Each patient was followed retrospectively and/or prospectively for 2 1/2 years with the study enrollment date defined as the date zidovudine therapy was begun.

USE OF COHORT STUDIES IN PHARMACOEPIDEMIOLOGY

Postmarketing surveillance studies are often cohort studies which have no clearly defined control group. Cohort studies in pharmacoepidemiology can evaluate: (1) the long-term effects of drugs; (2) effects which may be present only in very low frequency in a population; (3) effectiveness of drugs in customary practice, i.e., "the real world"; (4) efficacy of a drug for an indication for which the drug was not originally approved; and (5) modifiers of drug efficacy, e.g., concurrent medications, lifestyle, or severity of disease. In the pharmaceutical industry, postmarketing surveillance studies have sometimes naively been thought of as merely a way of monitoring adverse drug events. However, it is becoming increasingly apparent that pharmacoepidemiologic methods can contribute much more than the frequency of adverse drug events to studies of the utilization and effectiveness of drugs in various populations.

The number of persons exposed to a drug necessary to detect the true frequency of adverse drug events may be large. For instance, in order to have an 80% statistical power to detect an event that occurs once in every 5,000 patients, we would need to monitor a cohort of over 8,000 persons.[2] Thus, even though cohort studies are desirable over case-control studies, because bias can be more easily controlled in the former, they can be very expensive to conduct. Postmarketing surveillance methods utilizing large automated databases have allowed the monitoring of large cohorts without a simultaneous large increase in cost over case-control studies. As such, these cohort studies can permit us to calculate incidence rates in a subset of the population treated with a specific drug as compared to those not treated with the drug. We can determine incidence of adverse events as well as specific disease outcomes. This comparison can also be made in patients with the same disease, part of whom were treated with a particular drug, while part were treated with a different drug. Pharmacoepidemiologic studies can help us quantitate the effect of *confounding by the indication*, a type of bias which occurs when the indication for a specific drug therapy is associated both with treatment with that drug and with a higher probability of a given event. For instance, in patients with human immunodeficiency virus (HIV) infection, a fall in CD4+ lymphocyte (T4) count can be perceived as an indication for beginning antiviral therapy and also as a prognostic indicator for an adverse event, e.g., development of an opportunistic infection.

Some disadvantages of using large automated databases in postmarketing surveillance studies include problems associated with selection bias and questions of validity. For example, patients who are included in a population enrolled in a Health Maintenance Organization (HMO) in the United States are representative only of people who are working in the businesses which employ that particular HMO. Validity is not automatically extendible to individuals who are unemployed or working in other occupations. Of course, this is not a problem in countries where medical care is socialized, e.g., members of the Saskatchewan Health Plan, which includes nearly every Canadian citizen residing in that Canadian province. The utilization of large databases allows us to look both retrospectively and prospectively at drug exposure and outcome, thus reducing the need for long periods of time between the time a study is begun and the time data analysis is begun.

ILLUSTRATION OF A SUCCESSFUL COHORT STUDY

In classical epidemiology, we use certain well defined criteria to assess causality. These can be summarized as follows:
1.   Strength of the association
2.   Presence of a dose-response effect

3. Temporality, i.e., did the presumed cause precede the effect?
4. Consistency of the association
5. Specificity of the association
6. Biological plausibility

In cohort studies, especially because of their inherent risk of bias, as opposed to a randomized clinical trial, we often find it useful to apply these criteria to our results in assessing the likelihood that the hypothesized cause is related to the effect being studied.

As an example of a study which illustrates many of these important considerations in conducting a cohort study in a large population, let us look at a Japanese comparison of ionic and nonionic contrast media for radiologic studies. This was a nationwide comparative clinical study to examine the incidence of adverse drug reactions to two types of radiologic contrast media.[3] Prior to beginning the study, a one-month pilot study which included 17,187 cases tested the case record form to be used for the study. Certain items were eliminated and others were added so that the final form was a single page. It included a section for hospital code, date of exam, and patient code; another section with various patient data; a section for radiologic exam data; and a section on occurrence, symptoms, severity, and outcome of adverse drug reactions. The authors calculated that the necessary sample size was approximately 300,000 cases in order to have a β of 0.40, i.e., 60% power, to detect a difference at p=0.05 (2 tailed), on the assumption that the prevalence of severe ADRs to nonionic contrast media (1 per 14,000 patients) could be reduced to one-fourth of that seen with ionic contrast media. A total of 58 main hospitals and 148 affiliated hospitals were selected according to the minimum number of radiologic exams performed per month and in the anticipation that these hospitals would switch substantially from ionic to nonionic contrast media during the study period (approximately 2 years). The final number of cases collected was 352,817. Among these, 4.3% (15,170 cases) were excluded from analysis. The reasons for exclusions included that: (1) entries on the case record form were grossly incomplete; (2) radiographic examinations other than computed tomography (CT), intravenous urography, or intravenous digital subtraction angiography (DSA) were performed; (3) the contrast media used was not recorded; or (4) the presence or absence of an ADR was not recorded.

The overall incidence of adverse drug events among patients who received ionic contrast media was 12.66% compared to 3.13% in those patients receiving nonionic contrast media (Table 1). The odds ratio for this comparison was 0.22 (with confidence limits of 0.22 - 0.23), for a p-value of less than 0.01. The differences between patients receiving the two media were even greater when comparing severe or very severe adverse drug events in the two groups (Tables 1 and 2). One death was recorded in each group, but in neither case was death attributed to the contrast media used. When the frequency of adverse drug events was stratified according to age in the two groups, the rate of adverse drug events in patients receiving nonionic contrast media was lower in every age category (Table 3). When the dose-response effect was examined, again adverse reaction rates were higher among patients receiving ionic contrast media in every dose category (Table 4). When adverse reaction rates were compared to those seen in other studies of patients receiving the two types of media, results favored nonionic contrast media in every case (Table 5). The two groups were compared also according to underlying disease, injection mode, premedication, history of exposure to contrast media and associated adverse reactions, and history of allergy. In all comparisons, nonionic contrast media gave a profile which demonstrated a lower risk.[3] Original concerns in comparing these two contrast media had been that, while nonionic contrast media was expected to show a lower risk profile, it was unclear whether the decreased risk was substantial enough to justify the increased cost. From this study, the authors concluded that the risk of adverse events to ionic contrast media was so much greater than the risk associated with nonionic media, the higher cost of nonionic media was justified.

CONCLUSIONS

If an observational study is well designed, we will be able to apply the classical epidemiologic "tests" of causality. In this example of the comparison of two types of

Table 1.   Prevalence of ADRs

ADRs	Ionic Contrast Media (n = 169,284)		Nonionic Contrast Media (n = 168,363)		Odds Ratio of Nonionic to Ionic Contrast Media (95% Confidence Limits)[a]	
	No. of Cases	Prevalence (%)	No. of Cases	Prevalence (%)		
Total no. of cases	21,428	12.66	5,276	3.13	0.22[b]	(0.22-0.23)
Severe[c]	367	0.22	70	0.04	0.19[b]	(0.15-0.24)
Very severe[d]	63	0.04	6	0.004	0.10[b]	(0.05-0.19)
Death[e]	(1)	---	(1)	---	---	

a Odds ratio and 95% confidence limits calculated with the Mantel-Haenszel test.
b $P < .01$.
c Severe ADR defined as the presence of one or any combination of the following symptoms requiring some form of treatment: dyspnea, sudden drop in blood pressure, cardiac arrest, and loss of consciousness.
d Very severe ADR defined as a severe ADR that required the intervention of an anesthesiologist and/or hospitalization.
e In neither case was there a clear causal relationship with the contrast media used.

From: Katayama, Hitoshi et al. Adverse reactions to ionic and nonionic contrast media - A report from the Japanese Committee on the Safety of Contrast Media. Radiology 175: 621-628, 1990.

Table 2.   Severe ADRs

	No. of Cases	
Symptoms	Ionic Contrast Media (n = 367)	Nonionic Contrast Media (n = 70)
Dyspnea	204	50
Sudden drop in blood pressure	107	15
Loss of consciousness	4	0
Dyspnea and sudden drop in blood pressure	38	2
Dyspnea and cardiac arrest	1	0
Dyspnea and loss of consciousness	1	0
Sudden drop in blood pressure and loss of consciousness	12	3

From: Katayama, Hitoshi et al. Adverse reactions to ionic and nonionic contrast media - A report from the Japanese Committee on the Safety of Contrast Media. Radiology 175: 621-628, 1990.

contrast media, the *strength of the association* between nonionic contrast media and a lower adverse reaction frequency is shown in the comparisons of proportions of patients presenting with adverse reactions and in the significant odds ratios for the nonionic media cohort. When patients were stratified into six dose groups, a clear *dose-response effect* was seen in all but one category. In the dose group in which adverse reaction incidence was lower than expected, we can hypothesize that the size of the group (5-12 times the size of the other dose groups) may have contributed to this lower incidence. *Temporality* was assessed in the determination that 70% of adverse reactions occurred within 5 minutes of injection of the contrast media. The *consistency of the association* between lower toxicity and nonionic media was demonstrated by comparing the authors'

Table 3. Prevalence of ADRs by Age Distribution

Age of Patient (y)	Cases with Ionic Contrast Media			Cases with Nonionic Contrast Media		
	Total No.	No. with ADR (%)	No. with Severe ADR (%)	Total No.	No. with ADR (%)	No. with Severe ADR (%)
<1	272	2 (0.74)	0 (0)	916	4 (0.44)	0 (0)
1-9	2,701	338 (12.51)	2 (0.07)	5,479	138 (2.52)	4 (0.07)
10-19	6,359	1,068 (16.80)	26 (0.41)	7,066	319 (4.51)	5 (0.07)
20-29	8,842	1,615 (18.27)	21 (0.24)	8,009	372 (4.64)	5 (0.06)
30-39	16,428	2,806 (17.08)	49 (0.30)	14,569	661 (4.54)	6 (0.04)
40-49	25,352	3,825 (15.09)	69 (0.27)	23,386	962 (4.11)	13 (0.06)
50-59	40,311	5,025 (12.47)	69 (0.17)	38,014	1,200 (3.16)	15 (0.04)
60-69	38,807	4,087 (10.53)	82 (0.21)	38,220	996 (2.61)	10 (0.03)
70-79	24,807	2,185 (8.81)	41 (0.17)	26,201	507 (1.94)	8 (0.03)
≧80	4,681	371 (7.93)	6 (0.13)	5,562	81 (1.46)	4 (0.07)
No entry	724	---	---	941	---	---

From: Katayama, Hitoshi et al. Adverse reactions to ionic and nonionic contrast media - A report from the Japanese Committee on the Safety of Contrast Media. Radiology 175: 621-628, 1990.

Table 4. Prevalence of ADRs by Dose

Dose (mL)	Cases with Ionic Contrast Media		Cases with Nonionic Contrast Media	
	Total No.	No. with ADR (%)	Total No.	No. with ADR (%)
<20	4,139	916 (22.13)	8,401	334 (3.98)
21-40	17,286	3,235 (18.71)	13,585	652 (4.80)
41-60	11,135	1,824 (16.38)	7,940	411 (5.18)
61-80	3,684	736 (19.98)	4,994	247 (4.95)
81-100	103,231	11,681 (11.32)	120,792	3,024 (2.50)
>101	29,488	2,920 (9.90)	12,344	564 (4.57)
No entry	321	---	307	---

From: Katayama, Hitoshi et al. Adverse reactions to ionic and nonionic contrast media - A report from the Japanese Committee on the Safety of Contrast Media. Radiology 175: 621-628, 1990.

Table 5. Comparison of the Prevalences of Severe ADRs in Several Studies

Author (year)	Reference	Cases with Ionic Contrast Media			Cases with Nonionic Contrast Media		
		Total No.	No. with ADR	Prevalence (%)	Total No.	No. with ADR	Prevalence (%)
Katayama (1989)							
Severe	---	169,284	367	0.22	168,363	70	0.04
Very Severe		169,284	63	0.04	168,363	6	0.004
Palmer (1988)[a]	5	79,278	71	0.09	30,268	5	0.02
Wolf et al (1989)[b]	6	6,006	24	0.4	7,170	0	0
Schrott et al (1986)[c]	7	---	---	---	50,642	6	0.01
Shehadi and Toniolo (1980)[d]	4	214,033	106	0.05	---	---	---

a Severe ADR meant that urgent therapy and hospital admission were required; patient considered at risk.
b Severe ADR meant loss of consciousness, cardiac arrest, shock, or symptomatic cardiac arrhythmia.
c Severe ADR meant hospitalized treatment.
d Severe ADR meant that hospitalization was required. All cases in this study involved only intravenous urography.

From: Katayama, Hitoshi et al. Adverse reactions to ionic and nonionic contrast media - A report from the Japanese Committee on the Safety of Contrast Media. Radiology 175: 621-628, 1990.

results to results obtained in a number of other studies. *Specificity of the association* was not demonstrated for any single adverse reaction, but certainly a higher overall rate of adverse reactions was clearly apparent in the patients receiving ionic contrast media. The *biological plausibility* of the lower potential for adverse reactions to nonionic contrast media stems from the relative lower osmolarity of nonionic versus ionic media.

In summary, although cohort studies in pharmacoepidemiology can be expensive to conduct, they may be subject to less bias than are case-control studies. The ability to detect rare events may be limited by sample size. However, we have shown that a well designed study conducted in a large population can provide useful results. The reliability and validity of a pharmacoepidemiologic cohort study may well depend, however, on how well the study satisfies criteria for evaluating causal relationships.

REFERENCES

1. R. Moore, T. Creagh-Kirk, J. Keruly, G. Link, R. Chaisson and the ZVD-Epidemiologic Study Group, Long-term safety and therapeutic response in patients treated with zidovudine, *J Clin Res Pharmacoepidemiol.* 4:130 (1990) (Abstract).

2. D. L. Sackett, R. B. Haynes, M. Gent and D. W. Taylor, Compliance, *in*: "Monitoring for Drug Safety, 2nd ed." W. H. W. Inman, MTP Press, Lancaster, UK 471-483 (1986).

3. Katayama and Hitoshi et al., Adverse reactions to ionic and nonionic contrast media - A report from the Japanese Committee on the Safety of Contrast Media, *Radiology.* 175:621-628 (1990).

4. W. H. Shehadi and G. Toniolo, Adverse reactions to contrast media, *Radiology.* 137:299-302 (1980).

5. F. G. Palmer, The RACR survey of intravenous contrast media reactions: final report, *Australas Radiol.* 32:426-428 (1988).

6. G. L. Wolf, R. L. Arenson and A. P. Cross, A prospective trial of ionic vs non-ionic contrast agents in routine clinical practice: comparison of adverse effects, *AJR.* 152:939-944 (1989).

7. K. M. Schrott, B. Behrends, W. Clauss, J. Kaufmann and J. Lehnert, Iohexol in der ausscheidungsurographie: ergebinisse des drug-monitoring, *Fortschr Med.* 104:153-156 (1986).

USING RANDOMIZED TRIALS IN PHARMACOEPIDEMIOLOGY

Gordon H. Guyatt, M.D.

Department of Medicine
and Department of Clinical Epidemiology and Biostatistics
McMaster University
Hamilton, Ontario, Canada

Randomized trials are used in a variety of situations by the pharmaceutical industry. Whatever the context, the methodological rigor of the trial is crucial for valid results to be obtained, and for the conclusions of the trial to be accepted. In this paper, I will review the essential components of the randomized trial, and in the process will highlight some methodological issues which may be less familiar. I will then introduce a new way randomized trials are certain to find progressively more use by the industry, and that is in the conduct of systematic overviews, or meta-analyses. Finally, I will review the situations in which randomized trials have proved, or might prove, useful to the industry.

ESSENTIAL METHODOLOGICAL COMPONENTS OF RANDOMIZED TRIALS

Random Allocation

The primary limitation of studies (generally termed cohort studies) in which patients are allocated to treatment or control by methods other than randomization is that the determinants of outcome may not be distributed equally between groups. As a result, one cannot be sure if differences between groups are a function of the treatment received, or of an imbalance in prognostic factors. This would not be problematic if we were aware of, and could measure, all the relevant determinants of outcome. Under these circumstances, we could use statistical techniques to correct for any imbalance in prognostic factors. Unfortunately, there is no disease for which we understand the biology sufficiently well that we can, accurately and precisely, predict individuals' outcomes. The beauty of randomization is that it assures, if sample size is sufficiently large, that both known and unknown determinants of outcome are equally distributed between treatment and control groups.

It is worthwhile being aware of some more sophisticated aspects of the randomization process. Randomization is often stratified. By stratification, we mean that the randomization is constructed in a fashion that, within strata, patients are equally distributed between treatment and control arms. This is done by having a separate randomization schedule for each stratum. Ordinarily, within multicenter trials, one stratification variable is center. Thus, each center has a separate randomization schedule. Other stratification variables are chosen according to their power as predictors of outcome. For instance, if size of myocardial infarction is the best known predictor of outcome in a trial of post-myocardial infarction secondary prophylaxis, patients may be stratified according to whether their infarcts are large or small.

Drug Epidemiology and Post-Marketing Surveillance, Edited by B.L. Strom
and G. Velo, Plenum Press, New York, 1992

Particularly if there are a number of stratification variables, individual cell sizes may be quite small. For example, using the prior example, the cell composed of the patients in center 6 with small infarcts may be small. To ensure that a comparable number of patients receive active and control treatments, the randomization can be blocked. Blocking involves constructing the randomization so that after a certain number of patients (often 4 to 8) have been randomized, it is guaranteed that half will have been allocated to active treatment and half to placebo. The resulting balance across strata ensures that the two groups will be comparable with respect to major determinants of outcome, and also facilitates subgroup analysis in which the differential effect of treatments across strata can be explored.

Double-masking

Double-masking, or double blinding, is now a standard procedure in drug trials. Placebo medication must be identical in size, color, consistency, and taste to the active treatment. The fundamental purpose of double-masking is to minimize the likelihood of bias intruding on a number of possible fronts. First, the likelihood of systematic differential cointervention, that is management other than the experimental treatment, on the basis of group membership is minimized. Second, bias in the measurement of outcome is less likely.

The objectives of double-masking have often been viewed with considerable naivete. In the naive conception, the purpose of double-masking is to ensure that no one has any idea which patients are receiving active treatment and which placebo. In this naive conception, the effectiveness of blinding can be tested by asking participating physicians and patients to guess which treatment they are receiving. If their success rate is better than chance, some basic flaw in the masking process is suspected.

This logic ignores the fact that, to the extent a treatment is successful, trial participants receiving active treatment and their physicians will be more likely to correctly guess their allocation. Thus, a high successful guess rate can be a reflection of treatment efficacy, rather than a reflection of inadequate masking procedures. Side effects of treatment (such as bradycardia in patients with beta blockers) will also lead to a guess rate which is better than chance.

It follows from this that the appropriate way to conceptualize masking is as a process that introduces uncertainty. The introduction of this uncertainty decreases (but doesn't eliminate) the possibility of bias intruding. Perhaps fortuitously, the less effective the treatment in improving outcome, the more effective the masking process is likely to be.

Measurement of Outcome

The goal of rigorous measurement of outcome is to minimize both bias and random error. When bias acts in favor of the active treatment, it will spuriously increase the estimate of the effect size. When the measure of outcome is a continuous variable, random error will reduce the precision of the estimate of effect size. When the measure of outcome is dichotomous (dead or alive, myocardial infarction or no myocardial infarction), random error spuriously reduces the estimate of effect size.

The primary strategy for minimizing the biased assessment of outcome is blinding. Minimizing random error is achieved by precise definition of measures of outcome, standardization of measurement techniques, and testing and calibration to ensure reproducibility of measurement. In multicenter trials with dichotomous outcomes (disease-specific mortality, for instance), both bias and, particularly, random error can be reduced by a blinded review of whether an event has occurred. An adjudication committee handling this task will note instances in which classification errors have been made, and ensure their correction.

Analysis

There are two issues concerning analysis with which I would like to deal. The first is the need for an intention-to-treat analysis. The second is the issue of hypothesis testing versus estimation.

Intuitively, one might consider dropping patients who did not receive active treatment (for example, those whose compliance with treatment is poor) from the analysis. However, any analysis in which this is done is suspect. The reason is that those who do not comply may (unrelated to treatment) be systematically different, with respect to outcome, from those who do comply. As soon as one has different criteria applied to the treatment and control groups in who enters the analysis, the great advantage of randomization, comparability of treatment groups, is lost. Thus, investigators must live with the loss of power implicit in non-compliance with treatment. This suggests the importance of maximizing power by including only patients in whom compliance is likely to be high.

In considering and presenting the results of clinical trials, the traditional approach has been that of hypothesis-testing. A null hypothesis, that placebo and active drug are no different, is postulated. The trial is designed as an attempt to disprove this null hypothesis. This approach has a number of problems. First, trials are categorized as "positive" or "negative." This dichotomy is inevitably arbitrary. A trial that yields a p-value of 0.06 gives essentially the same message as one that yields a p-value of 0.04. Traditionally, however, the first trial would be viewed as negative, the second as positive. A second implicit deduction is that if a trial is positive the treatment should be administered, if negative it should not. Clearly, a positive trial in which the magnitude of effect was clinically unimportant would not mandate administration of treatment.

An alternative approach is that of estimation of the magnitude of effect. Here, the question is: "how big is the treatment effect" (one possible answer being zero). If one uses this framework, the result observed becomes the best estimate of treatment effect, and the confidence interval around this estimate tells us the possible range in which the true difference between active treatment and placebo lies. There is a very healthy trend away from hypothesis-testing and toward the estimation framework in evaluating and presenting the results of clinical trials.

Presentation of Results: Magnitude of Effect

In trials in which the primary outcome is a dichotomous variable, different strategies for presenting the magnitude of effect are available. The first is relative risk reduction, which is calculated by subtracting the incidence of the endpoint in the control group from the incidence in the treatment group, and dividing by the incidence in the control group. For example, if a drug reduces mortality from 10% to 5% the relative risk reduction is 50%; if the mortality is decreased from 10% to 7.5%, the relative risk reduction is 25%.

The problem with the relative risk reduction is that it does not capture the absolute magnitude of the impact of a new treatment. The reason is that this impact is proportional not only to the relative risk reduction, but also to the baseline risk. The baseline risk is not considered in calculating the relative risk reduction. For example, a drug that reduces mortality from 1 to 0.5% has the same relative risk reduction (50%) as one that reduces mortality from 10 to 5%. For any given number of patients treated, however, the impact of the second drug will be far greater.

The attributable risk reduction takes into account the baseline risk. The attributable risk reduction is the proportion of patients who would have had the event if untreated who are spared the event by receiving treatment. It is calculated by subtracting the incidence of the event in the treatment group from the incidence in the control group. If the incidence is 10% in the control group and 5% in the treatment group, the attributable risk reduction is 5%; if the incidence is 1% in the control group, and 0.5% in the control group, the attributable risk reduction is 0.5%. In both cases, the relative risk reduction is 50%.

The attributable risk reduction may be a difficult number for clinicians to intuitively grasp and use. Aside from attributable risk reduction, another way of including information about both the incidence and relative risk reduction in a single number is something called the "number needed to treat." The number needed to treat is calculated by dividing the number one by the attributable risk reduction, expressed as a proportion. The number needed to treat is interpreted as the number of patients to whom one needs to administer a drug to prevent a single adverse outcome event. For an attributable risk reduction of 5% (0.05), the number needed to treat is 20; for an attributable risk reduction of 0.5% (0.005), the number needed to treat is 200. This number is one that makes a lot of sense to clinicians, and is likely to see increasing use.

SCIENTIFIC OVERVIEWS

Scientific overviews, or meta-analyses, are likely to play an expanded role in the assessment of therapeutic efficacy. The rationale for meta-analysis is as follows. Any trial is limited by its sample size. That is, each trial is subject to the play of chance which will result in apparent effect sizes which differ from the true effect. Combining results from different trials effectively increases sample size, and should result in a more precise estimate of true effect than can be obtained from any of the individual trials.

Methodologic standards for evaluating scientific overviews are available[1], and are briefly summarized in Table 1. There are many controversial issues regarding the best way of conducting overviews. These include the best way of assessing validity and using validity assessments of the primary trials, the boundaries of what trials can be combined and what cannot, and the optimal statistical analyses. Nevertheless, meta-analyses have already made significant contribution to our assessment of treatment effectiveness, and will certainly be a more commonly used tool in the future.

THE USES OF RANDOMIZED TRIALS IN PHARMACOEPIDEMIOLOGY

For those in the pharmaceutical industry, the most obvious use of randomized trials is in so-called "pivotal trials." These trials are designed to convince regulatory agencies that a drug should be marketed. Their primary purpose is to demonstrate "efficacy"; that is, to show that the drug has a positive effect, in comparison to placebo, on an outcome that (it is generally agreed) is of some clinical importance.

There are other instances in which the pharmaceutical industry may find randomized trials of use. First, a drug may be licensed, but proof of efficacy for the most highly relevant endpoint may not be established. This would be true of most of the antihypertensive agents in use today; they have been shown to reduce blood pressure, but the evidence that stroke or myocardial infarction is reduced is indirect. A powerful example of this is a trial in which a number of antiarrhythmic drugs, previously licensed on the basis of their ability to suppress arrhythmias, were compared to placebo in patients with ventricular dysrhythmias following myocardial infarction[2]. The primary endpoint in this trial was sudden death. Unfortunately, two of the agents, encainide and flecainide, actually proved to increase the incidence of sudden death.

While randomized trials are of no use in finding out about rarely occurring side effects (the trials would have to be too long, and involve too many patients, for them to be feasible), they can be of use in determining the impact of frequently occurring side effects. This fact was appreciated by the manufacturers of captopril, an antihypertensive agent. In a post-marketing randomized trial, captopril was compared to a beta blocker and methyldopa, but the primary endpoint of the study was not blood pressure, but health-related quality of life[3]. The demonstration that patients taking captopril felt better than patients receiving the other agents provided the company with a very useful marketing strategy. The result of this experience is that other companies are now alert to the possibility of conducting studies of health-related quality of life after their drugs have appeared on the market.

A final use of randomized trials has to do with establishing the cost-effectiveness of new interventions. While of general interest in the industry, this has become particularly relevant in France. There, the price-setting process is based on the extent to which the company can demonstrate that their product makes an important new contribution to improving health. So-called "me too" products will be priced lower than truly innovative agents. Cost-effectiveness trials present special challenges. They include trying to simulate the real-world setting in which the drug will be administered ("management" or "pragmatic," rather than "explanatory" trials), and the measurement of total costs associated with alternative treatments and their associated outcomes.

Table 1.   Guidelines for Assessing Research Reviews

1)   Were the question(s) and methods clearly stated?
2)   Were the search methods used to locate relevant studies comprehensive?
3)   Were explicit methods used to determine which articles to include in the review?
4)   Was the validity of the primary studies assessed?
5)   Was the assessment of the primary studies reproducible and free from bias?
6)   Was variation between the findings of the relevant studies analyzed?
7)   Were findings of the primary studies combined appropriately?
8)   Were the reviewers' conclusions supported by the data cited?

REFERENCES

1.   A. D. Oxman and G. H. Guyatt. Guidelines for reading literature reviews, *Can Med Ass J*. 138:697-703 (1988).
2.   The Cardiac Arrhythmia Suppression Trial (CAST) Investigators, Preliminary report: effect of ecainide and flecainide on mortality in a randomized trial of arrhythmia suppression after myocardial infarction, *N Engl J Med*. 321:406-412 (1989).
3.   S. H. Croog, S. Levine, M. A. Testa, and et. al., The Effects of Antihypertensive Therapy on the Quality of Life, *N Engl J Med*. 314:1657-1664 (1986).

PHARMACOEPIDEMIOLOGY STUDIES USING LARGE DATABASES

Brian L. Strom, M.D., M.P.H.

Clinical Epidemiology Unit
Section of General Internal Medicine
Department of Medicine
University of Pennsylvania School of Medicine
Philadelphia, Pennsylvania 19104-6095

The study designs used in postmarketing drug surveillance are those used in epidemiology in general, including randomized clinical trials, cohort studies, case-control studies, case series, and case reports. Pharmacoepidemiology studies, however, represent unique applications of these, for three reasons.[1] First, randomized clinical trials are less likely to be useful, as they have already been conducted prior to marketing. Second, pharmacoepidemiology studies often must be performed very quickly, as pharmacoepidemiology questions frequently represent regulatory, commercial, and public health crises. Third, many of these studies require unusually large sample sizes. Because 500 to 3000 subjects are usually studied prior to marketing, a postmarketing surveillance pharmacoepidemiology study conducted as a randomized clinical trial, cohort study, or case series is generally unwarranted unless it can include at least 10,000 exposed subjects and, in the first two, another 10,000 controls. Analogously, a postmarketing pharmacoepidemiology case-control study must tap a population base of equivalent size.[2]

As an attempt to address these special issues related to pharmacoepidemiology, investigators have begun turning to large automated databases with medical data to conduct such studies.[3] There are a number of computerized collections of medical billing data which have been of use for such studies (see Table 1). The major source of these data is usually billing information (see Figure 1). When a patient visits a pharmacy and receives a drug dispensed for them, the pharmacy bills an insurance carrier, justifying that bill with the identity of the drug, the number of pills dispensed, etc. Similarly, when a patient visits a hospital or a physician for medical care, the hospital or physician bills the insurance carrier for the cost of that care, justifying that bill with the diagnosis or diagnoses under treatment. When these bills are submitted with unique identification numbers justifying the eligibility of the patient for insurance coverage, these pharmacy data, hospital data, physician data, and other possible data can be linked using these unique identification numbers and be available, therefore, for research purposes.

An example of a profile from one such database is represented in the Figure 2, as a demonstration of how this series of medical claims can provide insight into a patient's history. In this case, the patient is a 19-year old female with specified race and county of residence. The first column presented is the date, specified as a Julian date, i.e., the 226th day of 1980, the 54th day of 1981, etc. This format allows for easy calculation. The second column continues the diagnoses, coded by ICD-9-CM code. The third column includes drugs dispensed, recorded by National Drug Code. The fourth column presents the actual codes. The fifth column presents the strength or units of the drugs

Drug Epidemiology and Post-Marketing Surveillance, Edited by B.L. Strom
and G. Velo, Plenum Press, New York, 1992

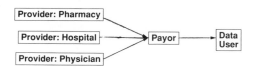

Figure 1.   Computerized Collections of Billing Data: Sources of Data.

Table 1.   Computerized Collections of Medical Billing Data

Program	Advantages	Disadvantages
Medicaid (e.g., COMPASS[R])	Size Ease of use Outpatient dxs	Skewed population No inpatient drugs Eligibility changes
Saskatchewan Health	Least skewed popn Prolonged history	Size Limited formulary Little outpatient data Dxs affect reimburs
Kaiser Permanente	Less skewed popn	Limited drug data computerized No outpatient dxs Limited formulary
Group Health	Less skewed popn Easiest access to medical records	Smallest No outpatient dxs Limited formulary

dispensed. The sixth column presents the provider identity number. This has two parts. The first part is an alphabetic code, which indicates the site of care. For example, an "I" code is a hospital discharge diagnosis, while an "X" code is a pharmacy claim. The second part of this code is an unique numeric code which identifies the provider himself or herself. The last column represents the quantity of drug dispensed. Thus, this young woman had an acute laryngitis in late in 1980 treated with a combination cold preparation and ampicillin. In early 1981 she had acute tonsillitis, treated with ampicillin. Two days later she experienced urticaria, treated with benadryl, possibly due to now a second exposure to ampicillin. In 1981 she had a fractured finger. Early in 1983 she had a pregnancy exam, with the pregnancy not yet confirmed. Three days later the pregnancy was still unconfirmed, but obviously suspected, since Bendectin[R] was prescribed. One week later the pregnancy was confirmed. Bendectin[R] and maternal vitamins continued. Months later she had threatened labor but did not actually deliver; the codes specified antepartum conditions, and they are not "I" codes, indicating hospitalization. A number of months later she subsequently delivered and then received postpartum follow-up care.

EXAMPLES OF LARGE DATABASES USED FOR PHARMACOEPIDEMIOLOGY RESEARCH

There are a number of computerized collections of medical data used for pharmacoepidemiology research (see Table 1). Data from some health maintenance

HEALTH
INFORMATION
DESIGNS, INC.

COMPASS SYSTEM
PATIENT DX/RX HISTORY PROFILE

PATIENT ID: 2000000**P   SEX: F   AGE: 19(1984)   COUNTY: 14   RACE: 2

DATE	DIAGNOSIS		DRUG		STRENGTH/UNIT	PROVIDER	QUANTITY
80226	ACUTE PHARYNGITIS	462				P-1304323	
80226		000074423	ORNADE SPANSULE			X-1304323	16
80226		000710402	AMCILL		250.000MG	X-1304323	28
81054	ACUTE TONSILLITIS	463				P-1338330	
81054		001722017	AMPICILLIN TRIHYDRATE		250.000MG	X-1042435	24
81057		000710471	BENADRYL		25.000MG	X-1062868	30
81057	URTICARIA NOS	7089				P-1062868	
81308		000710373	BENADRYL		50.000MG	X-1042435	20
81338	FX PHALANX, HAND NOS-CL	81600				0-2001052	
81338	FINGER INJURY NOS	9595				P-1157120	
81343	FX PHALANX, HAND NOS-CL	81600				P-1042435	
81364	FX PHALANX, HAND NOS-CL	81600				P-1054534	
82067	ABDOMINAL PAIN	7890				P-1157120	
82069	ABDOMINAL PAIN	7890				0-2001052	
82069	DYSPHAGIA	7872				P-1204767	
83025	JOINT PAIN-SHLDER	71941				X-1204767	
83025		000450414	TOLECTIN DS		400.000MG	X-1204767	21
83049	PREG EXAM-PREG UNCONFIRM	V724				P-1338330	
83052	PREG EXAM-PREG UNCONFIRM	V724				X-1338330	
83053		000680155	BENDECTIN			X-1370060	15
83061	PREG STATE, INCIDENTAL	V222				P-1370060	
83061		000055559	MATERNA 1-60			X-1338330	30
83070		000680155	BENDECTIN			X-1338330	15
83080		000680155	BENDECTIN			X-1338330	30
83110		000055559	MATERNA 1-50			X-1338330	30
83143	THREATENED LABOR NEC	6441				P-1157120	
83143	COMPL LABOR NOS-ANTEPART	65993				0-5171637	
83145		000055559	MATERNA 1-50			X-1338330	30
83192		000055559	MATERNA 1-60			X-1338330	30
83235	DIABETES-ANTEPARTUM	64603				P-1203877	
83245		000055559	MATERNA 1-60			X-1338330	30
83269	ACUTE PHARYNGITIS	462				P-1338330	
83274	ABN GLUCOSE TOLER-DELIV	64881				I-2001052	
83274	DEL W 4 DEG LACERAT-DEL	66431				I-2001052	
83283	ENLARGEMENT LYMPH NODES	7856				P-1338330	
83326	ROUT POSTPART FOLLOW-UP	V242				P-1370060	
84065	DISEASE OF PHARYNX NEC	47829				P-1304323	

Figure 2.   SAMPLE COMPASS PROFILE. (Reprinted, with permission, from Strom BL (ed)., Pharmacoepidemiology, New York: Churchill Livingstone, 1989, p. 176).

organizations can be very useful for this purpose. For example, Kaiser Permanente in Northern and Southern California each include more than 1 million patients.[4] The Oregon Kaiser plan includes between 300,000 to 400,000 patients. Each of these programs has centralized computerized hospital discharge diagnosis information which can be used to identify cases for case-control studies. However, the drug data that are computerized in these plans are limited. The outpatient pharmacies are completely computerized in Oregon, but only partly computerized in Northern and Southern California. In addition, there is no outpatient diagnosis information available except by chart review, and the formularies can be limited. Finally, these programs may not be large enough to address some important questions. Nevertheless, Kaiser Permanente, particularly in Northern California, has been used to perform some excellent pharmacoepidemiology studies.[4]

Group Health Cooperative of Puget Sound[5] is the health maintenance organization which has been used most often for pharmacoepidemiology research. This includes between 300,000 and 400,000 patients. It has a fully computerized pharmacy and easy access to medical records, making it an attractive source for such studies. However, it is the smallest of the computerized databases for pharmacoepidemiology research. Thus, it is only useful when both the drug and the disease are relatively common. In addition, it does not have outpatient diagnoses computerized and has a limited formulary. Nevertheless, it has been productive of much useful information.[5]

As another example, Saskatchewan Health[6] has billing data for the 1 million residents of Saskatchewan. It has a major advantage of being a large population-based system without the problems of changing eligibility that other insurance plans have. It has the major advantage of having a prolonged history, so that one can study long-term drug effects. However, its population is not as large as is necessary for some studies. Other limitations include: 1) a population with few blacks, 2) a large rural population, 3) a somewhat limited formulary, 4) limited outpatient data, and 5) potentially biased outpatient data, since reimbursement changes depending on the diagnosis. It has enormous promise and is beginning to be productive in pharmacoepidemiology.[6]

Finally, an alternative source of computerized billing data is Medicaid data.[7] Medicaid data can be particularly useful when very large sample sizes are needed or when outpatient diagnoses are needed. It can be used to conduct very large cohort studies or theoretically ideal case-control studies, drawing its cases from the large population and drawing a true random sample of population controls, avoiding one of the major limitations of case-control studies. However, Medicaid databases include data from a skewed population, skewed based on economic status, and do not include inpatient drug exposures. More importantly, it is difficult to differentiate between periods of good health and periods of ineligibility. Most significantly, important questions have been raised about the validity of the diagnosis data in these databases.

DISCUSSION

Thus, these large databases have a number of advantages (see Table 2). They can be very large, permitting one to perform studies of relatively uncommonly used drugs and relatively uncommon outcomes. They can be inexpensive to use, relative to the cost of performing an *ad hoc* studies of the huge populations included in these datasets. This is because the cost of data collection is borne by the administrative system which created the database. They are complete, including all medical care provided by any practitioner; one does not need to rely on patient recall or physician knowledge of care received by the patient from other physicians. They can population-based, allowing the calculation of incidence rates and the avoidance of selection bias. They can include outpatient drugs and diseases. Finally, and very importantly, they are not subject to recall bias or interviewer bias, as they do not rely on patient recall or interviewers to collect the data.

These databases also, clearly, have disadvantages (see Table 3). Most importantly, the diagnosis data in these databases must always be considered suspect, and so access to primary medical records must be obtained. There is no information available in the computerized database on some potential important confounding variables, e.g., smoking, occupation, alcoholism, etc. A few of the databases have direct access to patients to obtain this supplementary information, e.g., Puget Sound and Saskatchewan. Otherwise, studies must be limited to those which are not affected by these in a major

Table 2.   Computerized Collections of Medical Billing Data: Advantages

---

Size

Cost

Complete

Can be population-based

Can include outpatient drugs and diseases

No recall or interviewer bias

Table 3.   Computerized Collections of Medical Billing Data: Disadvantages

---

Cannot be used to performed randomized clinical trials

Incomplete information on potential confounders

Variable data elements

Outcome assessment usually cannot be quantitative, but simply present or absent

Uncertain data validity, especially for diagnoses

---

way. These databases only include illnesses severe enough to come to medical attention. Of course, these are the illnesses most likely to be important to study. Finally, some results may not be generalizable, e.g., information on health care utilization. Each of the databases contains its own skew. As noted, the Medicaid data are most skewed, by socioeconomic status. The health maintenance organizations tend to include a younger and healthier population of higher socioeconomic status, individuals who become eligible for their HMO coverage through their employer. Saskatchewan data are probably the most representative, but still may be atypical of other populations in the world. For this reason, one must be careful in generalizing descriptive data from these databases to elsewhere. Nevertheless, the use of homogeneous populations, e.g., Medicaid, can be useful in analytic studies, as one need not worry about confounding by socioeconomic status.

What are the uniquely useful and uniquely problematic situations for use of these databases? (see Tables 4 and 5.) Because of the large sample sizes available, these databases can be uniquely useful in the study of uncommon exposures and/or uncommon outcomes. Because of the absence of recall bias and interviewer bias, these databases can be particularly useful when one is studying outcomes most susceptible to such problems, e.g., perhaps birth defects. Because they can be population-based, these databases can be useful when a denominator is needed to calculate incidence rates. They are most useful when one is studying short-term drug effects, especially when these drug effects require treatment with specific drugs or specific surgical therapy. The latter can be used as markers of the outcome in question to validate the diagnosis data available. These databases are also very useful when one has objective, laboratory-driven diagnoses, easy to validate in the medical record. Finally, they are useful when one has limited time and a limited budget, as such studies can be performed more quickly and less expensively than *ad hoc* studies of many questions.

Table 4.   Computerized Collections of Medical Billing Data: Uniquely Useful
            Situations

The study of uncommon exposures and/or uncommon outcomes

When recall bias is a problem

When interviewer bias is a problem

Denominator needed to calculate incidence rates

Short-term drug effects, especially when they require specific drug or surgical therapy

Objective, laboratory-driven diagnoses

Limited time

Limited budget

Table 5.   Computerized Collections of Medical Billing Data: Problematic
            Situations

Illnesses which do not reliably come to medical attention

Inpatient drug exposures

Outcome poorly defined by ICD-9-CM coding system

Descriptive studies

Delayed drug effects

Important unknown confounders

Use of these databases is particularly problematic when studying illnesses which do not reliably come to medical attention, e.g., nausea, skin rashes, and headache. Ascertainment of these could well be incomplete. These databases do not have information on inpatient drug exposures. The databases are problematic when the outcome is not clearly defined by the ICD-9-CM coding system. For example, studies of Stevens-Johnson Syndrome are difficult, because this diagnosis is embedded in ICD-9-CM code 695.1, which also includes erythema multiforme, staphylococcal scalded skin syndrome, etc.[8] These databases are impossible to use to study an outcome like retroperitoneal fibrosis, as this diagnosis is embedded within a code for ureteral obstruction, and very little ureteral obstruction is likely to be due to retroperitoneal fibrosis.

These databases can be problematic when performing descriptive epidemiology studies, because of generalizability. They can be problematic in studying delayed drug effects, because of patient ineligibility. Finally, they can be problematic when there are important unknown confounders.

CONCLUSION

In conclusion, a number of different research resources are now available to perform pharmacoepidemiology studies. Each has advantages and disadvantages and each has been useful in certain situations. Included, more recently, are a number of medical databases derived from the billing process. The databases have the major advantage of being able to gather the large number of subjects necessary for pharmacoepidemiology studies quickly, efficiently, and relatively inexpensively. Because they are secondary data sources, however, none have all of the data one might want if one were gathering it de novo. Different compromises need to be made when using each. Careful attention to the relative strengths and weaknesses of each will allow an investigator to choose the optimal system to answer his or her pharmacoepidemiology question and the consumer of pharmacoepidemiology research to be aware of its limitations. It is unlikely that any single data source will ever fulfill all the diverse needs of this field. Certainly, none now does. The development of new systems of this type needs to be a high priority for the future.

REFERENCES

1.   B. L. Strom, Study designs available for pharmacoepidemiology studies, *in*: "Pharmacoepidemiology" B. L. Strom, ed., Churchill Livingstone, New York 13-26 (1989).
2.   B. L. Strom, Sample size considerations for pharmacoepidemiology studies, *in*: "Pharmacoepidemiology" B. L. Strom, ed., Churchill Livingstone, New York 27-37 (1989).
3.   B. L. Strom and J. L. Carson, Use of automated databases for pharmacoepidemiology research, *Epidemiol Rev.* 12:87-107 (1990).
4.   G. D. Friedman, Kaiser Permanente Medical Care Program: Northern California and Other Regions, *in*: "Pharmacoepidemiology," B. L. Strom, ed., Churchill Livingstone, New York 161-72 (1989).
5.   A. Stergachis, Group Health Cooperative of Puget Sound, *in*: "Pharmacoepidemiology," B. L. Strom, ed., Churchill Livingstone, New York 149-60 (1989).
6.   L. M. Strand and R. West, Health databases in Saskatchewan, *in*: "Pharmacoepidemiology," B. L. Strom, ed., Churchill Livingstone, New York 189-200 (1989).
7.   B. L. Strom, J. L. Carson, M. L. Morse and A. A. LeRoy, The Computerized Online Medicaid Analysis and Surveillance System: a new resource for post-marketing drug surveillance, *Clin Pharmacol Ther.* 38:359-64 (1985).
8.   B. L. Strom, J. L. Carson, A. Halpern, R. Schinnar, E. Sim, P. Stolley, H. Tilson, M. Joseph, W. Dai, D. Chen, R. Stern, U. Bergman and M. Shaw, Using a claims database to investigate drug-induced Stevens-Johnson Syndrome, *Stat Med.*, in press.

SCREENING FOR UNKNOWN EFFECTS OF NEWLY MARKETED DRUGS

Jeffrey L. Carson, M.D.
Brian L. Strom, M.D., M.P.H.

Division of General Internal Medicine
University of Medicine and Dentistry of New Jersey
Robert Wood Johnson Medical School
New Brunswick, New Jersey 08903
      and
Clinical Epidemiology Unit
Section of General Internal Medicine
Department of Medicine 19104-6095
University of Pennsylvania School of Medicine
Philadelphia, Pennsylvania

INTRODUCTION

Many new chemical entities were marketed throughout the world in the past decade. Since only limited information is available prior to marketing of a new drug, it is extremely important to monitor the safety of these drugs. The rapid detection of adverse drug reactions has important public health implications. Acute side effects occur in approximately 5% of patients taking a drug.[1] While most of these adverse drug reactions (ADRs) are mild and reversible (e.g., rashes, gastrointestinal distress), some cause significant morbidity and mortality. In addition, ADRs need to be detected, validated, and reported, so that clinicians can base a decision to administer a drug on known risks and benefits. While it probably unrealistic to think that any system might always avert tragedies such as the thalidomide episode[2], the hope is that it might detect such problems early enough to reduce the number of affected individuals.[3-7] Furthermore, new drugs need to be monitored for unknown beneficial effects.

Prior to marketing, new drugs are subjected to pre-clinical animal studies followed by three stages of clinical trials. However, pre-marketing trials are limited in their ability to identify drug effects. These limitations include[8,9]: 1) premarketing trials generally have fewer than 3,000 participants, so they cannot reliably detect rare drug effects (incidence less than 1 per 1,000); 2) premarketing clinical trials are of limited duration and therefore cannot detect long-term effects; and 3) the study population used in premarketing studies is often not representative of users of the drug, often omitting the elderly, patients with other co-morbid diseases, pregnant women, and children.

During the past decade ticrynafen, benoxaprofen, zomepirac, and suprofen, among others, were removed from the US market because of the discovery of serious ADRs presumably unknown at the time of drug marketing. The inability of premarketing studies to detect some important adverse reactions emphasizes the need for an effective system for screening drugs after marketing.

In this chapter we briefly review the methods that have been used to monitor for unknown effects of newly-marketed drugs. The primary focus of this discussion, however, will be a proposal for a new approach to this problem. The chapter will conclude

Drug Epidemiology and Post-Marketing Surveillance, Edited by B.L. Strom
and G. Velo, Plenum Press, New York, 1992

with a research agenda for future developments in this field. Much of the material presented here is based on material published previously.[10]

CURRENT APPROACHES

Spontaneous Reporting System

The spontaneous reporting system has been the foundation of postmarketing surveillance screening throughout the world. This system depends upon physicians, pharmacists, and other health care professionals to recognize an event as related to a drug, and then reporting it to a governmental agency (such as the US Food and Drug Administration), to the manufacturer, or in the medical literature. The possibility of a problem from a drug is suggested if a greater than expected number of reports of an adverse event is reported for a drug. This system is particularly useful when a drug commonly induces an otherwise rare disease.

The spontaneous reporting system has proven to be useful for screening for ADRs. During the past decade, the spontaneous reporting system was responsible for detecting serious problems in four drugs leading to there withdrawal from the United States market. Ticrynafen, a uricosuric diuretic, was reported in the medical literature to cause serious liver disease.[11,12] By the time of removal of the drug from the market in May 1980, the manufacturer had received 52 reports and the FDA had received four reports of hepatocellular injury from ticrynafen. Benoxaprofen (Oraflex[R]), a nonsteroidal anti-inflammatory drug, was withdrawn from worldwide use due to reports of 61 benoxaprofen-associated deaths in the United Kingdom.[13] Zomepirac (Zomax[R]), another nonsteroidal anti-inflammatory drug, was removed from the market because of reports of patients with anaphylactoid reactions first reported in the medical literature[14], and later confirmed in the FDA spontaneous reporting system files. The latest drug to be removed from the US market because of an ADR was suprofen (Suprol[R]), another non-steroidal anti-inflammatory drug. Suprofen's ADR (bilateral acute flank pain and reversible acute renal failure) was principally brought to the attention of the medical community by spontaneous reports to the manufacturer and FDA.

Despite these successes, the spontaneous reporting system has significant limitations.[15] The number of patients who are exposed to a drug is often unknown and the number of exposed patients who would have been reported if they had developed that adverse reaction is always unknown. Thus, it is impossible to calculate incidence rates. Without an incidence rate, one cannot determine whether the adverse outcome occurs more commonly than it would have been expected to occur spontaneously. In addition, the clinical importance of an ADR is difficult to determine without an incidence rate. Common reactions might warrant removing a drug from the market, while rare reactions would only require warning physicians. Under-reporting has also been a problem[16], despite the increasing number of reports in recent years.[17,18] Biased reporting is also a obstacle to the usefulness of this system. ADRs are reported more frequently with new drugs than with old drugs, with the greatest number of ADRs reported within two to three years after the release of a drug and increased reporting associated with publicity. Finally, the spontaneous reporting system is obviously unlikely to detect previously unknown beneficial drug effects.

Other Drug Event Systems

During the 1960s several groups systematically evaluated patients admitted to the hospital, searching for medical events caused by drugs.[19-26] The purposes of these programs were to describe drug utilization, to characterize ADRs and the patients at risk for ADRs, to determine the frequency of life threatening events, and to generate hypotheses about drug-induced disease. At least two very important observations have been made with these systems. The Boston Collaborative Drug Surveillance Program observed that aspirin use three months prior to admission to the hospital was associated with a significantly lower frequency of myocardial infarction.[27] This and other studies led to extensive work in this area, which has confirmed this very important finding.[28] Mitchell et al., by screening children in a neonatal intensive care unit identified that heparin flushes led to subdural hematomas.[29]

There currently are several systems which use outpatient cohort studies to monitor selected newly-marketed drugs. The best known is the Prescription Event Monitoring which was developed by Inman in 1982.[30-32] Copies of all prescriptions for drugs of interest are obtained from the United Kingdom's Prescription Pricing Authority and are used to identify patients in England who were prescribed the drug. Questionnaires are then sent to the prescribing general practitioner, requesting information on any clinical event that occurred since the drug was prescribed, as well as other relevant clinical information. Rates of events in patients exposed to the study drugs are then compared to those in patients exposed to other drugs or to the same patients before or after this drug exposure. An example of unexpected drug effects detected by this system while monitoring several nonsteroidal anti-inflammatory drugs, was that the rate of myocardial infarction increased when zomepirac was stopped.[33]

The Northern California Kaiser Permanente Medical Care Program has been used to screen for drug-induced cancer. Kaiser Permanente is the largest Health Maintenance Organization in the United States and has computer files on all members' hospitalizations. Friedman and colleagues have been observing the frequencies of new cancers in a large cohort of patients whose drug exposures were computerized in 1969-1973.[34,35] This system has been most useful in refuting hypotheses such as metronidazole's association with cervical cancer[36,37], digitalis being protective against breast cancer[38], and that rauwolfia derivatives cause breast cancer.[39]

Summary

The weight of the evidence suggests that the spontaneous reporting system has played a very important role in screening for ADRs. With the exception of the few examples presented, other systems have not made significant contributions. The limitations of spontaneous reporting systems cannot be overlooked. The absence of a control group, the lack of denominator data for calculation of incidence rates, and the presence of underreporting and biased reporting all dictate the need for the development of alternative or, more likely, supplementary systems.

PROPOSED SOLUTION

The ideal PMS screening system would have the following characteristics: 1) the ability to follow a large enough cohort of patients exposed to a new drug to detect important drug effects that occur less often than once in 1,000 exposed patients, and preferably even once in 10,000 individuals; 2) the ability to study a control group of unexposed patients; 3) the ability to study a control group of patients exposed to other drugs of the same class, if such drugs are available; 4) high quality exposure and outcome data; and 5) the ability to perform such studies at a reasonable cost. Table 1 outlines a proposed system. It is divided into hypothesis generating studies, hypothesis strengthening studies, and hypothesis testing studies.

Hypothesis Generating Studies

Study design. Postmarketing evaluation of a new drug should begin at the time the drug is marketed. A cohort of patients who receive the new drug should be identified and their experience followed. To determine if the new drug is associated with unexpected harmful or beneficial effects, it will be critical to use one or more comparison groups. At least three comparison groups are possible: 1) patients not dispensed a prescription to any related drug (unexposed), 2) patients dispensed, for the first time, another drug in same class as the study drug for the same indication; and 3) the same patient before and/or after receiving the study drug. The purpose of the first comparison group would be to determine if the drug is associated with any diseases, in general. The purpose of the second comparison group would be to examine whether the drug is associated with any diseases more or less frequently than other drugs of the same class. This information can be critical in determining the relative advantage or disadvantage of a drug in comparison to other therapeutic options available to the prescribing physician. The purpose of the third comparison group would be to use the same patient as the

Table 1. Proposed System for Postmarketing Screening of Newly Marketed Drugs

Design	Description
Hypothesis generating studies	
Cohort Studies	Cohort Accrual initiated at time of marketing of new drug
	Follow-up for multiple outcomes
	Associations submitted to signal algorithm
	Analysis repeated at predefined intervals
Case-Control Studies	Identify cases with disease that are commonly caused by drugs
	Compare antecedent drug exposure to that of a control group
	Associations submitted to algorithm
	Analysis repeated at predefined times
Hypothesis strengthening studies	
Cohort Studies	Conducted if signal generated by spontaneous reporting system
	Initiated at time signal is generated
	Uses entire experience of cohorts accrued during the signal generating study
	Follow-up only for outcome signalled by spontaneous system
	Provides incidence rates and relative risks
Case-Control Studies	Conducted if signal generated by spontaneous reporting system
	Initiated at time signal is generated
	Uses entire case group accrued during the signal generating study
Hypothesis testing studies	
Cohort Studies	Initiated to confirm signal
	Analysis includes control of confounding, dose-response, and duration-response
	Careful validation studies to verify diagnosis information
Case-Control Studies	Initiated to confirm signal
	Analysis includes control of confounding, dose-response, and duration-response
	Careful validation studies to verify exposure and diagnosis information

control, to control for patient-specific factors while exploring new symptoms which developed before or after exposure to a drug.

For a meaningful contrast between these groups, it is important that the comparison groups are similar to the exposed group in all ways except the exposure to the drug of interest. In general, this will be difficult to assure with the first two types of control groups, since the populations of patients in the different groups are likely to have some differences. This is the principal reason to use the third type of control group. To minimize these differences when using the first two control groups, the cohorts should atleast be matched for variables such as age and sex. In addition, patients exposed to other drugs in the same class might be matched for the number of different drugs in that class dispensed during the preceding year, or both groups restricted to the first prescription of a drug in that class. This is important because patients using other drugs in the same class are likely to be different than those receiving their first prescription for a drug of that class. For example, patients switched from one drug to another in a class may have had an adverse reaction to another drug of the same class. Because this methodology is intended for screening (hypothesis generating) purposes, more definite control for other potential confounders is not performed until subsequent analyses, which are carried out only if signals are generated. If available, the use of four matched controls per exposed patient in each comparison group will optimize the trade off between the study's statistical power (i.e., its ability to detect signals early) and its cost.

A comprehensive system should also screen for the teratogenic effects of newly-marketed drugs. A subgroup of women who were pregnant at the time of accrual into the index cohort would be compared to pregnant women in the two comparison groups, again matched for age. Once the appropriate cohort has been identified, the infants' records can be followed at regular (e.g., three month) intervals for a period of approximately one year or more, for a diagnosis of a birth defect.

There are four categories of outcomes that should be considered: 1) diseases suspected of being associated with the drug of interest based on animal studies, premarketing clinical studies, and previous studies of drugs in the same class; 2) diseases which have frequently been associated with drugs, for example hematologic, hepatic, allergic, dermatologic, neurologic, and renal disorders; 3) aggregates of birth defects which make teratologic sense; and 4) all other diseases except for the primary indication for the study drug. Any analysis must only examine incident cases, that is a disease which occurs for the first time after drug exposure, in order to be more certain that it is drug-induced disease.

Analysis. To explore possible associations between the new drug and the outcomes described above, the incidence of the diseases of interest in the cohort of patients exposed to the new drug would be compared to the incidence in each of the comparison groups. This would be performed by calculating incidence density ratios with confidence intervals and p-values. Incidence density ratios are similar to relative risks, but adjust for unequal follow-up. A person-time methodology is used because of varying lengths of follow-up within the comparison cohorts. The p-values would be one-sided (90% confidence intervals) when testing for outcomes associated with the drug based on prior evidence. Tests for all other outcomes would be two-sided (95% confidence intervals).

These analyses would be repeated at regular intervals, for example every three months. As the number of patients exposed to the new drug increases, the ability of the analysis to detect associations will increase. In addition, this type of analysis permits comparisons across time periods to examine if the results remain consistent. Cohort accrual and analysis continues until the accrued sample size is large enough to detect or exclude a risk of specified magnitude.

Signal generating studies for newly-marketed drugs should begin as soon as the drug is released. Data relating to subsequent medical events then becomes available over time. Statistical analyses should be performed using all data available at any point in time, in order to maximize the chance of detecting an important drug-induced risk quickly. However, the performance of multiple statistical tests over time can increase the chance of falsely finding an elevation in risk, such that the true risk of finding a falsely positive study is greater than the nominal alpha level chosen for each test.[40] In addition, if one examined 100 medical events to see if they are associated with use of a drug, then using an alpha level of 0.05 one would expect five of the analyses to be statistically significant purely by chance. This could be addressed in the usual fixed sample design by adjusting the alpha level using Bonferroni's correction.[41] This procedure divides the alpha level of 0.05 by the number of comparisons (in this case dividing 0.05 by 100, yielding an alpha level of 0.005). However, this procedure results in a lower power to detect associations, which is problematic, given the purpose of this analysis is early detection.

To address the problem of multiple testing of accumulating data, we could use group sequential methods of analysis. Group sequential methods allow for repeated significance testing of data accumulated over time while maintaining a required overall level of significance.[42,43]

Sequential analysis can be applied to postmarketing surveillance, where one is exploring whether a specific drug increases the risk of a particular adverse event. To apply group sequential methodology, one must first specify the number of looks at the data that are planned. As an example in postmarketing surveillance, consider a monitoring plan where one compares an accumulating cohort of exposed patients to a control cohort including unexposed individuals or individuals exposed to another drug. Data could be examined, say, every three months for a maximum of four years, for a total of 12 analyses. If insufficient data are available at the onset or at any given 3 month period, the analysis would be delayed until adequate data has accumulated, prolonging the period of surveillance.

We must also stipulate the number of patients in both the exposed and control cohorts to be compared at each look. If insufficient data are available at any given 3 month period, the analysis would be delayed until the next 3 month period. Under the assumption that we are testing for drug effects which occur shortly after a new drug is taken (an anaphylactic reaction is a clear example), it is reasonable to define the outcome to be a medical event occurring within at most three months after the first administration of the drug. Hence, the outcome of each patient (event vs. no event) is known prior to the collection of data from the next bolus. This restriction enables the calculation of the resulting true alpha and beta values for the sequential testing procedure.[43]

A different approach from the one above is to use survival analysis to study outcomes associated with long-term drug use.[44] Large cohorts of exposed and unexposed patients could be followed sequentially, with multiple testing performed on all available data up until experiencing the event. The outcome variable of interest would be time until developing the ADR. The "survival" experience of the groups would then be compared.

Finally, a further modification is warranted if we want to simultaneously look at multiple medical events potentially arising from the use of particular newly-marketed drugs. Suppose there are five classes of medical events to be monitored and we perform the above group sequential method test for each of these outcomes separately. The probability of falsely rejecting the null hypothesis of no elevation in risk again becomes inflated because of the multiple testing. We could account for this by applying the Bonferroni correction.[41,45] This is done by dividing each outcome-specific alpha by the number of tests done.

Disease-specific screening studies. An alternative and complimentary approach to screen for unknown drug effects is to perform a series of case-control studies. This technique would be useful for diseases which are commonly caused by drugs or where the outcome is very rare (case-control studies are more efficient than cohort studies for very rare diseases. In addition, this approach could be used to screen older drugs and/or those not specifically subjected to the cohort approach. Cases would be defined as diseases which are commonly caused by drugs, such as renal, liver, dermatologic, allergic, hematologic, and neurologic disease. Four controls per case would be randomly chosen from the remaining population and antecedent drug exposures would be compared. Each case-control study would be repeated at regular intervals. The number of cases would increase over time, permitting more sensitive studies. The analysis would use similar techniques to adjust for multiple comparisons and sequential testing, as described for cohort studies.

Hypothesis-Strengthening Studies

Hypothesis-strengthening studies refer to analyses that are performed to further examine hypotheses identified from another source, such as the spontaneous reporting system, or generated from the cohort or case-control screen described above.

Signals arising elsewhere. If the spontaneous reporting system detects a signal, or a signal is generated based on premarketing animal or clinical data, or based on experience with another drug, then the index cohort and comparison groups can be used to corroborate or refute these signals. Specifically, such a methodology would complement the spontaneous reporting system by: 1) inexpensively and efficiently either substantiating or repudiating signals generated by the spontaneous reporting system, and 2) providing additional information, such as incidence rates and relative risks, not accessible via the case reports of the spontaneous reporting system--statistics which are crucial in making clinical and regulatory decisions. This information can then also be used to guide the decision about whether to perform additional scientific studies. In addition, since government agencies are often forced to make regulatory decisions before definitive studies are performed, this information can be used to assist this process as well. Rapid access to this information could tremendously aid difficult regulatory decisions that must be made quickly.

At the time of a signal from the spontaneous reporting system, one could immediately examine the cohorts that have already been accrued. The entire sample size accrued to the point that signal is received would be utilized to study the association. The specific outcome to be studied will be dependent on the signal generated via the spontaneous reporting system. To examine incident cases, members of the original cohort who had the outcome of interest prior to the time of cohort accrual would be removed from the cohort for this analysis. Rather than conducting analyses at three month intervals as described for signal generation, one analysis would be conducted, using the total experience of the cohorts accrued through the time of the signal. Because we would be exploring a specific drug/disease association rather than multiple outcomes, it would not be necessary to address the problem of multiple comparisons. Therefore all data could be pooled and a p-value of 0.05 used to indicate a statistically significant association. Of course, the available sample size would be constrained by the number of patients who used the study drug from the time of marketing until the time the signal was noted.

Signals arising from the proposed screening procedures. Hypotheses generated from the cohort or case-control screening methodology above must be examined further by controlling for potential confounding variables and exploring dose-response and duration-response relationships. Analyses would be performed similar to those which would be performed in hypothesis testing studies. However, since such hypotheses arose from the same data and were not *a priori* hypotheses, these analyses cannot be considered as testing hypotheses and further corroboration would be required from other data. Of course, one would also explore biological plausibility, as well as whether there is consistency in the findings obtained with other clinically related outcomes (e.g., whether results are similar with both emphysema and chronic bronchitis).

Hypothesis Testing Studies

Hypothesis testing studies involve examining a hypothesis generated from some other source. The identical procedures would be followed as in the preceding section.

Because of the very large sample sizes that are required to carry out these screening procedures, record-linkage systems are probably the only realistic approach to this problem.[44,46] Record linkage refers to the ability to bring together computerized information about an individual, for example, information on drug use and diagnoses, from different sources.

Illustration

To illustrate the preceding principles, we describe a study screening for previously unknown effects of a newly marketed angiotensin converting enzyme (ACE) inhibitor. ACE inhibitors are commonly prescribed drugs for the treatment of hypertension, and congestive heart failure. We will call our new agent drug Z.

At the time of introduction of drug Z into the US pharmaceutical market, we would initiate a study using a cohort design. The exposed group would be defined as those patients dispensed drug Z. Five control groups would be used. The first four would be: 1) patients who are not exposed to any ACE, 2) patients exposed to ACE 1 and not drug Z, 3) patients exposed to ACE 2 and not drug Z, and 4) patients exposed to ACE 3 and not drug Z. These comparison groups would be used to determine if the new drug is associated with a medical event, in general, and whether this disease occurs more frequently (or less frequently) in patients exposed to the new drug than other drugs of the same class used for similar indications. The comparison groups would be matched to the study group for age and sex, with 4 controls of each type for each exposed subject. Patients will be restricted to those receiving their first prescription for the drug of interest. Finally, the fifth control group will be the same patients who received drug Z, exploring their history prior to receiving it.

Outcomes would be defined as the occurrence of a disease of interest within 30 days after each prescription one of the ACE, and during the time periods in the unexposed group identical to when patients in the exposed group received drug Z. Three categories of outcomes would be considered. The first would include aggregates of ICD-9-CM diagnoses representing diseases suspected to be associated with exposure to drug Z, based upon animal studies, pre-marketing studies, and studies of other drugs of the same class. These might include neutropenia, renal failure, anaphylactic reactions, and chronic cough. The second group would include groupings of ICD-9-CM diagnoses representing diseases which have frequently been associated with drugs, e.g., liver disease, erythema multiforme, phototoxicity, or fetal abnormalities. The final group will be all ICD-9-CM codes, analyzing each separately.

The next step in planning this study is to determine the number of boluses of data that one wishes to examine. This will depend upon the number of patients that will receive the drug, and the urgency of detecting an ADR. The fewer the number of boluses of data one examines, the lower the critical value (i.e., the easier it is to demonstrate statistical significance), but the longer it may take to detect an ADR. We would suggest using 12 boluses of data over a 3 year period.

Next one needs to determine the number of outcomes to examine. Suppose that, in premarketing studies, concerns were raised about the hematological and renal toxicity of drug Z. Therefore, this screening procedure will focus on neutropenia, anemia, thrombocytopenia, and acute renal failure, and nephrotic syndrome. With five outcomes of interest, we will use an alpha level of 0.01 (0.05 divided by 5, as per the Bonferroni correction), and a beta level of 0.1.

We would also examine diseases which have frequently been associated with drugs and all ICD-9-CM codes separately. However, these outcomes would have to be interpreted very cautiously because of the multiple statistical tests that would be performed. Any associations found could be considered only a hypothesis which might warrant further investigation.

FUTURE DEVELOPMENTS

Before such a system could be implemented, significant statistical development is necessary. Our analysis limits the number of outcomes to five. This is likely to be inadequate in many situations. One might want to screen for hundreds of potential medical events for each drug. For this many comparisons, the Bonferroni correction produces statistical tests of very little power. Yet, correction is still necessary if one wants to limit the number of false positive signals. Therefore, other approaches need to be developed.

This system must also be tested. This might best be done by attempting to replicate recently discovered unexpected effects of drugs and to see if it might have detected the problem before the spontaneous reporting system detected it. It would need to be used with several new drugs to see whether it functioned as designed.

Computer development would be needed so that this process could be automated as much as possible. This might include providing incidence density ratios or odds ratios adjusted for some common confounding variables and automated removal of patients with a prior history of an outcome so that only incident cases are examined.

When both the regulatory agencies and drug companies are faced with a crisis related to a drugs safety, they usually do not have adequate time or data to make an appropriate decision. The spontaneous reporting system may suggest a problem, but without incidence data, appropriate control group, nor a comparison group of other drugs in the same class used for similar indications it is often impossible to make an informed decision. The development of a system such as that described above has the potential to provide the necessary information to make a decision which protects the public against a potentially dangerous drug while protecting the investment of the drug company as well as the use of the drug for patients in the future.

REFERENCES

1. H. Jick, Adverse Drug Reactions, in: "Topics in Pharmacology and Therapeutics," R. F. Marone, ed., Springer Verlag, New York 397 (1986).
2. J. L. Schardein, ed, "Chemically-Induced Birth Defects," Marcel Dekker, New York, 215 (1985).
3. J. L. Carson and B. L. Strom, Techniques of postmarketing surveillance: an overview, Med Tox. 1:237 (1986).
4. A. Goldberg, Drug Safety - The role of doctors, pharmaceutical companies and the medical press, Br J Clin Prac. 39:5 (1985).
5. D. H. Lawson, Post-marketing surveillance in the UK (1984), Br J Clin Pharmacol. 22:71S (1986).
6. F. M. Lortie, Postmarketing surveillance of adverse drug reactions: problems and solution, Cand Med Assoc J. 135:27 (1986).
7. P. D. Stolley, and B. L. Strom, Evaluating and monitoring the safety and efficacy of drug therapy and surgery, J Chron Dis. 39:1145 (1986).
8. J. Idanpaan-Heikkila, A review of safety information obtained from phases I, II, and III clinical investigations of sixteen selected drugs, Rockville, MD: Food and Drug Administration, Center for Drug and Biologics, 1 (1983).
9. R. J. Temple, J. K. Jones, and J. R. Crout, Adverse effects of newly marketed drugs, N Engl J Med. 300:1046 (1979).
10. J. L. Carson, B. L. Strom and M. L. Morse, Screening for Unknown Effects of Newly Marketed Drugs, in: "Pharmacoepidemiology," B. L. Strom, ed., Churchill Livingstone, New York (1989).
11. P. Bolli, F. O. Simpson, and H. J. Waal-Manning, Comparison of tienilic acid with cyclopenthiazide in hyperuriceaemic hypertensive patients, Lancet. 2:595 (1978).
12. M. Lakin, Joggers liver, N Engl J Med. 303:589 (1980).
13. Committee on government operations: Deficiencies in FDA's regulation of the new drug "Oraflex." House Report 1:98-511 (1983).
14. S. A. Samuel, Apparent anaphylactic reaction to zomepirac (Zomax), N Engl J Med 304:978 (1981).
15. G. A. Faich, International drug surveillance, Drug Info J. 19:227 (1985).
16. J. M. Leiper, and D. H. Lawson, Why do doctors not report adverse drug reactions, Neth J Med. 28:546 (1985).
17. W. H. W. Inman, The United Kingdom, in: Monitoring for Drug Safety, W. H. W. Inman, ed., MTP Press, Lancaster 36 (1980).
18. J. T. Nicholls, The Practolol Syndrome - A Retrospective Analysis, Postmarketing Sruveillance of Adverse Reactions to New Medicines - Medico-Pharmaceutical Forum, Publication No. 7:4 (1977).
19. M. G. MacDonald, and B. R. Mackay, Adverse drug reactions, Experience of Mary Fletcher Hospital during 1962, JAMA. 190:115 (1964).

20. L. G. Seidl, G. F. Thornton, J. W. Smith, and et. al., Studies on the epidemiology of adverse drug reactions, III. Reactions in patients on a general medical service, *Bull Johns Hopkins Hosp.* 119:299 (1966).

21. R. I. Ogilvie, and J. Reudy, Adverse drug reactions during hospitalization, *Canad Med Assoc J.* 97:1450 (1967).

22. N. Hurwitz, and O. L. Wade, Intensive hosptial monitoring of adverse reactions to drugs, *Br Med. J.* 1:531 (1969).

23. H. Jick, O. S. Miettinen, S. Shapiro, and et. al., Comprehensive drug surveillance, *JAMA.* 216:467 (1971).

24. S. Shapiro, D. Slong, G. P. Lewis, and et. al., Fetal drug reactions among medical inpatients, *JAMA.* 216:467 (1971).

25. G. J. Caranasos, R. B. Stewart, L. E. Cluff, Drug-induced illness leading to hospitalization, *JAMA.* 228:713 (1974).

26. M. Levy, H. Kewitz, W. Altwein, and et. al., Hospital admissions due to adverse drug reactions, A comparative study from Jerusalem and Berlin, *Eur J Clin Pharmacol.* 17:25 (1980).

27. Boston Collaborative Drug Surveillance Program, Regular aspirin intake and acute myocardial infarction, *Br Med J.* 1:440 (1974).

28. The Steering Committee of the physicians' health study research group: Preliminary report: findings from the aspirin component of the ongoing physician health study. *N Engl J Med.* 388:262 (1988).

29. S. M. Lesko, A. A. Mitchell, M. F. Epstein, and et. al., Heparin as a risk factor for intraventricular hemorrhage in low birth weight infants, *N Engl J Med.* 314:1156 (1986).

30. W. H. W. Inman, Postmarketing surveillance of adverse drug reactions in general practice, I: Serach for new methods, *Br Med J.* 282:1131 (1981).

31. N. S. B. Rawson, and W. H. W. Inman, Prescription Event Monitoring: Recent experience with 5 NSAIDs, *Med Tox.* 1(Suppl 1):79 (1986).

32. W. H. W. Inman, Prescription Event Monitoring: A preliminary study of benoxaprofen and fenbufen, *Acta Med Scand.* (Suppl) 683:119 (1984).

33. W. H. W. Inman, N. S. B. Rawson, and L. V. Wilton, Prescription - event monitoring, *in:* "Monitoring for drug safety, 2nd ed.," W. H. W. Inman, ed., MTP Press Limited, Lancaster 213 (1986).

34. G. D. Friedman, and H. K. Ury, Initial screening for carcinogenicity of commonly used drugs, *J Natl Cancer Inst.* 65:723 (1980).

35. G. D. Friedman, and H. K. Ury, Screening for possible drug carcinogenicity: a second report of findings, *J Natl Cancer Inst.* 71:1165 (1983).

36. C. M. Beard, K. L. Noller, W. M. O'Fallon, and et. al., lack of evidence for cancer due to use of metronidazole, *N Engl J Med.* 301:519 (1979).

37. G. D. Friedman, Cancer after metronidazole (Letter), *N Engl J Med.* 302:519 (1989).

38. G. D. Friedman, Digitalis and breast cancer (Letter), *Lancet.* 2:875 (1984).

39. G. D. Friedman, Rauwolfia and breast cancer: no relation found in long-term users age fifty and over, *J Chron Dis.* 36:367 (1983).

40. P. Armitage, C. K. McPherson, and b. C. Rowe, Repeated significance tests on accumulating data, *J R Statistic.* 132:235 (1969).

41. D. F. Morrison, Multivariate Statistical Methods, 2nd ed., McGraw-Hill, New York 33 (1976).

42. S. J. Pocock, Group sequential methods in the design and analysis of clinical trials, *Biometrika.* 64:191 (1977).

43. B. S. Pasternak, and R. E. Shore, Group sequential methods for cohort and case-control studies, *J Chron Dis.* 33:365 (1980).

44. B. S. Pasternak, R. E. Shore, Group sequential methods for cohort and case-control studies, *J Chronic Dis.* 33:365 (1980).

45. F. M. Lortie, Postmarketing surveillance of adverse drug reactions: problems and solution, *Canad Med Assn J.* 135:27 (1986).

46. J. K. Crombie, The role of record linkage in post-marketing drug surveillance, *Br J Clin Pharmac.* 22:77S (1986).

HOSPITAL DATA SOURCES

Judith K. Jones, M.D., Ph.D.

Georgetown University
and The Degge Group, Ltd.
Washington, D.C.

PURPOSE

This paper addresses the hospital as a site for pharmacoepidemiology studies, particularly with respect to the development and use of automated data. A brief history of efforts to develop automated data in this site will be presented, followed by an example of one data base, and, finally, descriptions of the types of studies which have been or could be carried out. The advantages and limitations of these studies and the resources will be outlined to point out needs for future development in this part of the discipline.

HISTORY

Place of Hospital Surveillance in Overall PMS

Although a considerable amount of drug use occurs in the hospital setting, it is still limited, as illustrated in Figure 1, to a much smaller proportion of the market of drug

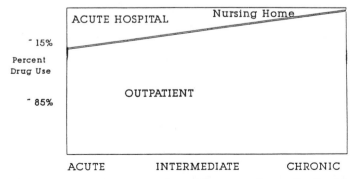

Figure 1.   A diagrammatic representation of the approximate distribution of inpatient and outpatient drug use. Depending upon how estimates are made, the precise proportion in the sectors varies.

Drug Epidemiology and Post-Marketing Surveillance, Edited by B.L. Strom
and G. Velo, Plenum Press, New York, 1992

use, roughly 15% of the total drug market dollar volume. Further, the potential range of drug effects is more limited, since the duration of exposure for any given individual is short and acute effects are usually the only ones of interest. Nonetheless, certain types of drugs, notably intravenous antibiotics and analgesics, are used only in this setting. The information about their actual use outside of clinical trials is limited, so there is clearly need for more detailed information.

Ironically, the opportunity for much more detailed observation of potential drug effects is offered in this setting, but this is often confounded by the fact that many events are crowded into the average 5-7 day length of stay. There are many other drugs, dozens of laboratory tests, and various therapeutic procedures. The patient enters either acutely ill, or undergoes surgery, and rapidly changes, usually toward return to health, over hours and days. Because of the large number of events, including drug administrations occurring in multiple sites, it has been quite difficult to obtain accurate data on drug exposure in this setting. Only a limited number of hospital automated data sources including drug data have been developed. The logistic requirements and difficulties with developing such resources will be explored here.

History of Data Base Development - The Predominance of Hospital Studies

Postmarketing observational drug studies were first carried out in the hospital setting, most likely because of the apparent advantages of having patients in a structured setting and available for interview, with data already being gathered. These early studies did not rely upon automated data, although the information collected was later entered into a computer, as in the case of the Boston Collaborative Drug Surveillance Program.[1]

FDA Interest

In fact, one of the early interests in developing automated collection of data within the hospital setting came from the FDA Division of Drug and Biological Experience, which had the mission of collecting information about the use of and problems with drugs after marketing. Studies of drug use had been quite possible for drugs used in outpatients, because of the existence of:

1. The IMS America data bases on outpatient prescriptions, which provided through one data source (National Prescription Audit[2]) an estimate of the number of new and refilled prescriptions dispensed in retail pharmacies for outpatients.
2. The IMS NDTI, or National Disease and Therapeutic Index, a physician-based audit of prescribing which described the reason for prescribing a drug in a particular person. Although this included some inpatient prescribing, it has not been considered as a representative sample of inpatient drug prescribing or use.
3. The Prescription Data Service, a separate patient-based audit of the prescribing of new and refill outpatient prescriptions, carried out by Prescription Card Services.[2]

No comparable source of information existed for the hospital setting, except: 1) the IMS National Hospital Data Audit, which only collected data on package and kilogram sales to hospitals, and 2) the data on total kilogram sales of each approved New Drug Application product which FDA regulations required manufacturers to provide on a periodic basis. Neither gave very good estimates of exposure per individual, although some attempts were made to use the European-based DDD (defined daily dose) methodology to estimate individual antibiotic exposure within the hospital setting[3]. Therefore, when serious questions arose, such as the concern over benzyl alcohol as a preservative in multi-dose vials used for injection, or Vitamin E used in injection, the need to develop an ongoing resource to record *patient-specific drug exposure information* in the hospital was recognized.

Thus, articles were written[4,5] and a pilot project initiated by FDA to stimulate the development of such a resource in the private sector. It was recognized, especially after initiating the pilot project, that the development of such a resource was a major undertaking on a similar scale to that of IMS America's outpatient drug audit, and that the capability of the FDA to carry out this was beyond the scope of its budget and mandate. This pilot project was carried out in two hospitals, comparing patient-based drug exposure information derived from pharmacy profiles to medical records. It revealed several important points which are covered more extensively in a recent discussion of this area:[6]

1. It is very difficult to capture the total drug exposure for any given patient within the hospital setting, because it occurs at a number of different sites (hospital bed, radiographic suite, surgery suite) and is controlled by different people (pharmacy, nursing station, radiology, surgery, and anesthesiology).

2. No one part of the medical record provides an accurate summary of the *total* drug exposure. Drugs given while the patient is in his/her bed are recorded on the floor; those given in surgery are recorded in the operating record; those given in recovery are recorded in the recovery room record; and those given during radiographic or other procedures are recorded in the procedure note (or not at all). In an intensive care setting, where many events may occur within an hour in a severely ill patient, it is very unlikely that all drug administrations are recorded. This was specifi-cally demonstrated in the case of attempts by the Centers for Disease Control and FDA to identify the extent of saline flush administrations in neonatal intensive care units in follow-up of the benzyl alcohol problem. Intravenous flushes of saline were not always recorded (CDC-personal communication, 1983). This finding even extended to narcotics, where careful recordkeeping is mandatory.

3. The recording of other information which would facilitate an adequate "drug profile" for monitoring of drug-related events is also quite variable, and confounds the goal of collecting relevant information on this topic. For example, weight, height, and blood type are not consistently found on hospital records. Further, a recent study of drug history taking in the hospital has continued to indicate highly variable and incomplete data.[7]

Although this pilot study pointed out the difficulty of the endeavor and did not result in pursuit of the specific methodology used, in addition to the already existing marketing study resources which regularly carry out ad hoc audits of use of particular products, several efforts did arise at about this time which could address this need for hospital-based data. It is unclear whether these new efforts related in any way to the regulatory interest, since many pharmaceutical manufacturers, also using the outpatient data, saw the need for a comparable inpatient-based resource.

RECENT EFFORTS

In the 1980's two very similar sources of hospital-based drug information linked to patient diagnosis, procedures, and outcome developed almost in parallel, and a third developed as a pilot project which is now amenable to widespread use.

The Medimetrik and IHS Data Bases.

The first two, MediMetrik and IHS, now the Walsh Hospital Drug and Diagnostic Index developed in the last half of the 1980's, with the objective of creating true record linkage of drug use to all major events in the hospital. They were developed by linking several diverse data sets which are commonly gathered and computerized in the U.S. hospital setting. Those hospitals which had computer systems collecting *all* of the following were eligible for inclusion in the system:

Administrative data. These data, including patient identification, demographics, insurance, admission-discharge dates, and disposition, are routinely collected on all patients hospitalized in acute care hospitals.

Pharmacy profile data. In some hospitals, computer systems have been developed to profile the medication history of an individual patient, typically using data from the unit dose distribution systems on the hospital floor combined with original drug orders. This is a pivotal part of the hospital record linkage system, since each dose had to be linked, in time, to a given patient. Thus, any system based on maintenance of a stock of drugs on the floor for as-needed use, as was once commonly the case, would not allow for this careful record of drug exposure in an automated fashion.

Pharmacy drug purchase system. This file, maintained by the pharmacy for use in inventory and purchasing of drugs, also maintains price data, which can be linked to individual profiles for estimation of drug costs/hospital stay.

Medical records computer system. The primary and secondary diagnoses and all procedures and complications are routinely collected in a standardized form for computerization.

Approximately 50 hospitals provided data to each of these data base "managers," who worked with the individual hospitals to link the different data sets into a coherent comprehensive data base which profiled the entire hospital stay for an individual patient. Thus, each dose of each pharmaceutical entity, including over-the-counter drugs and any other agents dispensed by the pharmacy, were captured and, depending upon the accuracy of the unit-dose system, could be recorded along with the time and dose administered. This would be linked to the procedures by day (procedures being a major activity in the hospital setting) and the discharge diagnoses (up to 20 ICD-9CM codes).

An example of a typical printout of such a profile is shown in Figure 2. In the case of Medimetrik, the data were collected from 50 hospitals which were, while the data base was operating (through 1988), representative of the U.S. national hospital surveys[8] and thus were able to provide an estimate for national inpatient use of pharmaceuticals. Several audits of these data were published and some studies, as yet unpublished, were carried out. Unfortunately, the Medimetrik source was discontinued, partly due to the monumental difficulty of maintaining the quality control of the tremendous amounts of data generated within *each* hospital. If one considers that, for a typical patient with a 7-day length of stay receiving 10 different pharmaceutical products, at least 40 different dosings/day would be recorded, along with 10-20 different diagnoses, 4-10 different procedures, and at least 10 other descriptors of demographic, outcome, diagnosis-related group (DRG), and financial status. Maintenance of the quality and coherence of each file at each site in each of many hospitals is a large task, particularly if the original data collection is not necessarily standardized!

The other effort, IHS, collects similar data, although it has had limited use except for FDA internal estimates of hospital drug use and in-house pharmaceutical marketing use, and no specific pharmacoepidemiological studies have been produced.

It is important to emphasize that the lack of such work may be less a statement of the inadequacy of the effort than of the actual difficulty in developing a *stable, quality-controlled* record-linkage data resource for ongoing use.

Ironically, hospitals around the U.S. and elsewhere have long had an interest in automation of services, and for over twenty years, certain functions have been maintained on computer data bases. However, almost invariably, the purpose of these automation efforts have been to streamline either financial or logistic management and, thus, data has not necessarily been collected in such a way to facilitate studies of patients by any medical or pharmaceutical groupings. Thus, hospital pharmacies and hospital central supply areas have often had useful automated *inventory* data systems to assist in monitoring supply of products. Given the variety and short stay of individual patients, the value of data on individuals in such systems is small. Similarly, the availability of automated laboratory systems in U.S. hospitals has been commonplace for a number of years, and these *have* been patient-based. However, given the volume of data and the *privacy* of the information, the notion of integrating this with any other data system in a hospital has often been rejected, until recently. Accordingly, the U.S. hospital environment has commonly been one where automation has been accepted for management, but not for health care or public health purposes.

```
MEDIMETRIK                                                      PAGE    1
            DIAZ   DIAGNOSES AND THERAPY REPORT
REQUEST ID: TEST001  SEQ: 740 HOSP: 0022 205037  -861202      RUN ON 03/24/88
     HOSP SIZE:                 REGION:

CASE DATA
  DRG: 107 CORONARY BYPASS W/O CARDIAC CATH    SPECIALTY: UNSPECIFIED OUTLIER: NO
  AGE/SEX: 63 MALE   RACE: OTHER   SERVICE: CARDIOLOGY
  ADMIT TYPE: EMERGENCY   SOURCE: EMERG. ROOM   DIS STATUS: HOME
  ADMITTED: 12/02/86   DISCHARGED: 12/12/86   DRUG COST:   $435.45
  PAYOR: BLUE CROSS          LOS: 10 DAYS

  DIAGNOSES                          PROCEDURES          PERFORMED ON DAY
  413.9 ANGINA PECTORIS NEC/NOS      36.13 AORTOCOR BYPAS-3 COR ART   4   P
  414.9 CHR ISCHEMIC HRT DIS NOS     88.56 CORONAR ARTERIOGR-2 CATH   2   P

DRUG USAGE                                                    -- DAY OF STAY ---
DRUG               STRENGTH/PACKAGE  FORM RT MFG       DOSE   DOSES THERAPY 1234567890 1234567890
                   SCHED START-STOP                                  DAYS

MANDOL        15130  CEPHALOSPORIN
                     3:00- 5:23   VIAL IJ LILLY     200 MG    6     3     X X X
                     3:00- 4:00        IJ           200 MG    1     1     X

ROBINUL-FORTE 23100  ANTISPAS. SYNTHETC
                     3:00- 3:00   TABS OR ROBINS       -      1     1         X

EPHEDRINE SULFATE 28120  BRONCHO GEN.OTH
             50 MG/ML  4:00- 4:00   SOLN IJ ABBOTT    50 MG   1     1         X

NEO-SYNEPHRINE 31600  CARDIVASCUALR AGENTS
             1 %    4:00- 4:00  1 ML SOLN IJ WINTH-BRE  .1 ML  1     1         X

ALBUMINAR 5   53521  NTML SERUM ALBUMIN
             250 ML   6:00- 6:00   SOLN IJ ARMOUR   250 ML    1     1              X

FERROUS GLUCONATE 48110  HEMAT.IRON ALONE
             300 MG   6:00- 6:23   TABS OR UPSHER   300 MG    3     6     X X X X X   x
             300 MG   6:00- 10:23       OR          300 MG    5     5     X X X X X   x
             300 MG  11:00- 11:23       OR          300 MG    2     1

HEPARIN SODIUM 11200  ANTICOAG. INJECT
             1,000 U/ML  4:00- 4:23  VIAL IJ LYPHOMED  1 U/   2     1     X
HEPARIN SODIUM 1,000 U   4:00- 4:23  SYRN IJ WYETH IV  1 U/   2     5
             1,000 U   7:00- 10:23              IV     3 UU   3     4     X X X X   x
             1,000 U   7:00- 11:00              IV     3 UU   1     1
HEPARIN SODIUM 1,000 U  11:00- 11:00  SYRN IJ WYETH IV  1 U   1     1
HEPARIN SODIUM 5000 U  10:00- 4:00   SYRN IJ WYETH IV  1 U   1     6         X
```

Figure 2.   An example of a typical MEDIMETRIK Drug Profile of a hospitalized patient.

87

At least one major exception to this has resulted in a unique, diversified, and potentially very useful automated "record linkage" system that has been developed in one hospital to a very considerable extent, and is being exported as a commercial system to other hospitals. This is the "HELP" system, developed at the Latter Day Saints Hospital in Salt Lake City, Utah. This system was developed recognizing the need to coordinate the many automated systems already extant, to facilitate both hospital and medical management. Accordingly, the system has evolved into a very diversified tool for managing many types of information: patient, specialty, and function-based. Figure 3

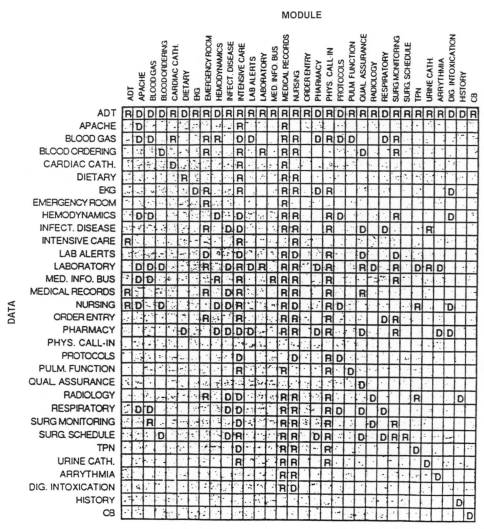

Figure 3.   A matrix of data elements and outputs from the Latter Day Saints Hospital HELP system.[9] An "R" indicates the 'module' uses the 'data' in the creation of HELP system Reports. A "D" indicates the 'module' uses the 'data' in the HELP system Decision logic.

illustrates a matrix of the information modules and uses currently being applied. Incidentally, the system is viewed as useful for postmarketing drug surveillance, and some papers describing this have appeared.[9]

CURRENT STATUS OF HOSPITAL DATA SOURCES

Automated

Other than the data relating to kilogram purchases of drugs by hospitals, currently, the only multi-hospital source of automated record linkage inpatient data is available from Walsh Hospital Drug and Diagnostic Index.

Non-automated

A number of ad hoc efforts to collect drug-related data in the hospital setting have been developed for both commercial and research purposes. For targeted, specific questions, these have worked well and may represent the most efficient method to answer some specific types of questions. For example, Dr. T. Grasela and colleagues at the University of Buffalo, using a network of clinical pharmacists in a variety of hospitals, have been able to carry out a number of studies.[10] Although the older Boston Collaborative Drug Surveillance Program of hospital surveillance has been discontinued, it has been activated more recently in two sites to carry out a specific study of a muscle relaxant, atricurium, although the divergent results in the two sites underline the many variables that likely affect the assessment of use of drugs in a hospital setting.[11,12]

EPIDEMIOLOGIC STUDIES OF HOSPITAL-BASED DRUG EFFECTS

For certain types of drug effects, a small or moderate number of hospitals can be surveyed on an ad hoc basis for occurrence and/or rates of relatively common effects, and this approach has been utilized by a number of researchers, cited above. However, there is also a need by both regulatory agencies and manufacturers to have an understanding of the larger, public health scope of overall drug use and exposure in the hospital setting. Since the approximately 6000 acute care hospitals in the U.S. vary widely with respect to many characteristics (number of beds, private vs. public, teaching vs. non-teaching, urban vs. rural) which affect drug use, it is much more difficult to obtain a representative sample from which national estimates of drug exposure can be made. Accordingly, for estimation of person-based drug exposure alone, there is a need for this type of data, since most estimates are currently made based on either kilograms purchased, or market sample surveys.

Further, there is also a need for multi-hospital record linkage data sources which are based on standardized data collected in a standard manner. Extension of either the IHS or HELP system to a wider range of hospitals may make this possible in the foreseeable future.

For these or related record linkage data bases to be used for retrospective epidemiologic studies of drug effects in the hospital setting, however, there will be some continued limitations for some types of studies, but not all. Studies of events which are measured by discrete, unambiguous outcomes marked by objective measures in a hospital chart, such as death, intubation, initiation of specific therapy (intravenous glucose, intravenous anticonvulsant) will be relatively amenable to study, with careful planning. Many events, however, will be much more difficult to study because of several factors:

1. The events, such as respiratory arrest, are typically confounded by one or more factors;
2. The recording of findings, particularly in progress notes and patient history and physicals, is highly variable and non-standardized;
3. Many events, such as gastrointestinal bleeding in an ill, older person, will have many potential causes, which may never be defined, despite access to an entire medical record.

4.   Many events, as in outpatient records, are seldom or incompletely detected and/or described. Depression and incontinence, as well as even postural hypotension, are cases in point.

Thus, as in the outpatient setting, epidemiological study of drug associated events can be facilitated by the availability of automated, linked data which describes these populations of patients. These data will certainly assist overall surveillance and help generate hypotheses of potential problems, but will vary in usefulness with the questions addressed and, until totally automated hospital records are available, with the quality of the data collected in that setting.

REFERENCES

1.   R. R. Miller and D. J. Greenblatt, "Drug Effects in Hospitalized Patients," J. Wiley & Sons, New York, pp 1-27 (1976).

2.   J. K. Jones and D. L. Kennedy, Data sources and methods for ascertaining human exposure to drugs, *J Toxicol Clin Toxicol*. 21:237-251 (1984).

3.   D. L. Kennedy, M. B. Forbes, C. Baum, and J. K. Jones, Antibiotic use in U.S. hospitals in 1981, *Am J. Hosp Pharm*. 40:797-801 (1983).

4.   M. B. Forbes, L. B. Burke, and J. K. Jones, Need for uniform data elements in hospital drug use review, *Am J Hosp Pharm*. 38:711-715 (1981).

5.   C. Baum, M. B. Forbes, D. L. Kennedy, and J. K. Jones, Patient drug profiles and medical records as sources of hospital drug use information, *Am J Hosp Pharm*. 40:2191-2193 (1983).

6.   J. K. Jones, Hospital Data Bases;, in: "Pharmacoepidemiology," B. Strom, ed., Churchill Livingstone, New York, NY. pp. 213-227 (1989).

7.   M. H. Beers, M. S. Munekata, M. Storrie, The accuracy of medical histories in the hospital medical records of elderly persons, *J Am Geriatr Soc*. 38:1183-1187 (1990).

8.   National Center for Health Statistics, Acute Hospital Survey (1985).

9.   R. S. Evans, R. A. Larsen and J. P. Burke, Computer surveillance of hospital acquired infections and antibiotic use, *JAMA*. 256:1007-1011 (1986).

10.   T.   Grasela,   A   Nationwide   Drug   Surveillance   Network,   *in*: "Pharmacoepidemiology Vol. I," S. Edlavich, ed., Lewis Publishers, Chelsea, MI. pp. 171-189 (1989).

11.   H. Jick, B. Andrews, H. H. Tilson and et. al., Atricurium-A Post Marketing Surveillance Study: Methods and U.S. Experience, *Br. J. Anesth*. 62:590-595 (1989).

12.   D. H. Lawson, G. M. Paice, R. J. Glavin and et. al., Atricurium-A Post Marketing Surveillance Study: U.K. Study and Discussion, *Br. J. Anesthes*. 62:596-600 (1989).

HOSPITAL-BASED INTENSIVE COHORT STUDIES

Keith Beard, B.Sc., M.B.

Consultant Geriatrician
Victoria Infirmary
Glasgow
United Kingdom

Before discussing recent experience with intensive hospital based drug monitoring systems, it is appropriate to consider the relevant historical background. The idea that treatment of any kind may be harmful as well as beneficial is not new and has been with us for many years.[1] The qualitative assessment of treatment associated risk is well encapsulated in the long established maxim "primum non nocere." This translates roughly as "the most important thing is to do your patients no harm," which is roughly equivalent to the idea that the chance of benefit from treatment should outweigh the risk of an adverse outcome. This sounds a self-evident concept but for it to operate properly it must be based on scientific fact and, sadly, this has not always been the case.

Before the discovery of useful drug therapy, many useless (with hindsight) treatments were meted out for severe and life-threatening conditions, for example, outdoor treatment for pneumonia, cold bath treatment for typhoid fever, water deprivation for cholera, or insulin-induced hypoglycemia for schizophrenia. The fact that these treatments themselves carried a serious life-threatening risk was really irrelevant as most of the diseases which they were supposed to treat carried a fatal or very serious outcome anyway. In the first half of the twentieth century, there were few drugs of established efficacy, and for the few that were available, risks associated with treatment were thought to be quite acceptable. Typical examples were mercury treatment for syphilis or digitalis treatment for heart failure.

The situation has changed rapidly and dramatically in the second half of the twentieth century for a number of reasons. The scientific method of assessing treatment and outcome has become universally established and rigorously necessary. There has been a rapidly expanding number of available drug treatments and, as that began to happen, there were isolated case reports and anecdotes of adverse drug reactions (ADRs). One of the earliest attempts at quantification of ADRs was the assessment of chloramphenicol-induced aplastic anemia, when 408 cases reported over a 12-year period were described in detail.[2] However, it was the so-called thalidomide disaster of drug-induced phocomelia which provided the major stimulus to the development of drug monitoring systems in the early 1960s.[3] These included the development of spontaneous reporting systems, but the limitations of these systems were recognized from an early stage. In 1965 Finney advocated a more rigorous approach to the assessment of ADRs.[4] He suggested that it ought to be possible to record all demographic and clinical information on hospitalized patients together with information on all clinical events, whether or not these events were thought to be related to drug treatment. He perceived that detailed analyses of the results of such data gathering might lead to the detection and quantification of previously unsuspected adverse drug effects.

Drug Epidemiology and Post-Marketing Surveillance, Edited by B.L. Strom
and G. Velo, Plenum Press, New York, 1992

In 1966, Cluff and colleagues reported work done in 1964 in Baltimore from what was essentially the very first intensive monitoring program.[5] In 1969, Hurwitz reported monitoring work done in 1965/66 when she had collected all the clinical information herself in the medical wards of a British hospital.[6] In 1966 Jick and Slone started the pilot scheme that was to become the Boston Collaborative Drug Surveillance Program (BCDSP).[7] The methods used by the BCDSP have been described in detail elsewhere.[8] Briefly, nurse monitors collected routine demographic social and medical information from consecutive admissions to hospital. Details of drug exposures before the hospitalization were obtained from patients by the monitors using a standardized interview conducted shortly after admission. Details of all drug exposures during the hospitalization were also recorded using standardized forms. The monitors attended ward rounds where they gathered information concerning undesired or unintended events thought by the attending physicians to be related to drug therapy. The degree of certainty that any event was causally related to drug therapy was assessed by the attending physician and at a later date by an independent clinical pharmacologist. In addition, information on certain specific events occurring during hospitalization was recorded routinely, whether or not these events were thought to be due to drug therapy. The resulting data were rigorously checked to ensure accuracy, completeness, validity, and consistency. Data were stored in computer files for subsequent analyses. After the pilot scheme, the BCDSP was expanded to operate in medical wards in six different countries and, by 1976, information had been collected from over 50,000 medical inpatients.

The aims and objectives of the BCDSP were similar to those of other groups using this method of surveillance, and these included the study of:

1. Patterns of drug use in hospital.
2. Acute adverse drug reactions occurring in hospital as a result of in-hospital drug use.
3. Serious or life threatening events or adverse drug reactions.
4. Pre-hospital drug use and associations between that and diseases or events at the time of admission.

The BCDSP has been, undoubtedly, the most successful of the intensive inpatient monitoring programs and it is, therefore, appropriate to review their work in some detail.

BCDSP STUDIES

Drug Utilization Studies

Drug utilization was not one of the principal aims of the program but routine review of the data produced co-incidentally some interesting findings. One example showed a marked difference in drug use patterns between patients monitored in Scottish hospitals as compared with patients monitored in American hospitals.[9] Seven hundred and twenty-one Scottish patients used an average of 4.5 drugs per admission, whereas 1,442 American patients used more than twice as many. Differences were found for somatic conditions such as diarrhea or dehydration and also for specific conditions such as diabetes and hypertension. More ADRs were noted in American patients, but this increase was commensurate with overall increased drug use. There was a constant drug-specific ADR rate in both countries.

Marked differences in intravenous fluid therapy were noted both between countries and within countries. The frequency of intravenous fluid therapy reached 54% in one American hospital, whereas in three hospitals in Scotland, Israel, and Canada it was no higher than 8%. Two Scottish hospitals in one city showed a marked difference, despite the fact that patients were well matched, both demographically and by disease type. Bias seemed unlikely and it was thought that there was a genuine difference in prescribing habits between the two hospitals. Of particular note in this study was the observation that 15% of intravenous fluid recipients developed an adverse effect directly related to fluid therapy.[10]

Descriptive Studies

Descriptive studies published by the BCDSP since 1966 cover many different areas. Drug-related deaths among medical inpatients were not thought to be a common occurrence and it was valuable to have this consistently quantified in different countries.[11] In this study, only 24 drug-attributed deaths were found among 24,462 consecutive medical admissions. Cytotoxic drugs, intravenous fluids, and digoxin were responsible for two thirds of these, but it was noted that many of these 24 patients were seriously ill and may have died anyway. In only 6 of the 24 cases was it thought that the drug-attributed death could have been prevented.

One of the earliest studies in 1968 reported the association between anticoagulant therapy and bleeding.[12] After only 97 heparin recipients had been monitored, an association was found between bleeding and therapy, particularly in females and in those over the age of 60 years. This ability to identify sub-groups of patients at particularly high risk has been a real strength of the program. In 1980 a much more detailed review of anticoagulant-associated bleeding was published.[13] Various predictors of bleeding were identified, including sex, dose, morbidity, previous aspirin use, previous alcohol use, and possibly age and renal function. In this study it was noted that the 7-day cumulative risk of bleeding during heparin therapy was 9%.

Routine review of the data resulted in the publication of a number of factors found to be associated with the short-term effects of the then commonly used hypotensive drug methyldopa.[14] Of 26,294 monitored patients, 1,067 received methyldopa during hospitalization and, of them, 10.3% experienced hypotension to a clinically significant extent. The frequency of hypotension was found to be associated with age (young more so than old), renal function, weight, dose of drug, and admission blood pressure. In addition, sub-groups showed marked associations, e.g., patients with renal impairment receiving a high dose were much more likely to suffer hypotension compared to those with normal renal function receiving a low dose. This was an exciting and important type of study for, from an observational base, it produced results that were both biologically and pharmacologically plausible. Furthermore, the adverse effects were found to be occurring during every day clinical use of a commonly used drug and the results suggested that, by paying attention to the various predictors, dose could be adjusted accordingly and the chance of sustaining an adverse effect could be reduced.

Hypothesis Testing Studies

It was possible to test independently generated hypotheses using the large body of data gathered by BCDSP. In many cases the data were very suitable for this because they were gathered by researchers and monitors who, during the time of data gathering, were unaware of hypotheses likely to be tested subsequently. Bias, therefore, was unlikely.

The relationships between ADRs and biochemical data was one area where hypothesis testing was successfully carried out. For example, the anticonvulsant drug phenytoin was found to be more toxic when the serum albumin concentration was low, the rate being 11.4% when albumin was less than 30 g/l and 3.8% when the albumin concentration was greater than 30 g/l.[15] This relationship was found to be independent of age, dose, and renal function. The hypothesis under test was confirmed, namely, that because phenytoin is both strongly protein bound and of a low therapeutic index, a reduction in protein concentration leads to an increase in free drug concentration and hence toxic effects.

In a similar way a hypothesis concerning the interaction between phenytoin and the anti-tuberculous drug isoniazid was tested. The overall ADR rate for phenytoin, was found to be low at 3%, but the neurological toxicity of phenytoin, manifesting as drowsiness, confusion, or cerebellar dysfunction, was found to be as high as 27% when the drug was administered in conjunction with isoniazid. This hypothesis had been suggested in case reports and the likely explanation was competition for protein binding sites between the two drugs, but the hypothesis had not been formally tested until this work was published.[16]

A further example of hypothesis testing was that of the effect of smoking on increased drug metabolism. Smoking might be expected to increase drug metabolism as smoking can induce hepatic microsomal activity. This was tested by comparing the frequency of drug-induced drowsiness in smokers and non-smokers.[17] In benzodiazepine users, drowsiness was less common in heavy smokers than non-smokers and this effect was not seen in phenobarbital users. The detailed hypothesis was that cigarette smoke stimulates the metabolism of drugs that are not themselves powerful enzyme inducers.

Hypothesis Generating Studies

With such a large body of information available for study, it was clearly sensible to conduct regular reviews of the data to see if any information about previously unsuspected ADRs might be uncovered. Review of the data in this way resulted in the publication of information regarding drug-induced gastrointestinal bleeding when a variety of drugs were implicated.[18] Of particular note was the observation that the powerful loop diuretic agent ethacrynic acid could cause gastrointestinal bleeding. Furosemide, a diuretic of comparable potency and with a similar mechanism of action, was not associated with bleeding. This side effect was not suspected by the attending physicians in individual cases and the hypothesis was only generated after a large body of data was reviewed, although a previous finding had been noted with intravenous administration of the drug.[19] Other drugs found to be associated with bleeding included heparin, steroid, aspirin, warfarin, and very many others in small numbers.

Pre-Hospital Drug Use

Recording drug intake in the period leading up to hospitalization was not a particular strength of the program, as it relied on patient recall over a three month period. This information was, however, recorded as accurately as possible and a number of interesting studies emerged from this part of the database. Hospital admissions due wholly or in part to adverse drug effects numbered 260 (3.7%) out of 7,017 monitored patients. The most commonly implicated drugs were digoxin, aspirin, steroids, warfarin, and guanethidine, with small numbers of many other drugs making up the total. This figure of 3.7% is in agreement with other studies and, although there were only small numbers of cases associated with individual drugs, the total number of drug-related admissions formed a significant fraction of the total number of admissions.[20]

Review of pre-hospital drug use from a hypothesis generating point of view yielded the observation that there was a significantly lower mortality in aspirin users than in non-users. Detailed analysis showed this to be due to a lower incidence of myocardial infarction.[21] The work was repeated two years later on a larger group of patients with similar results.[22] The association was found in patients with a wide variety of primary diagnoses and, although various potential risk factors for myocardial infarction such as diet and exercise were not known, it seemed unlikely that these could have caused significant confounding. This work generated considerable excitement but, coming as it did from an observational database, the information was not thought strong enough to indicate that prevention with aspirin was truly worthwhile. It was many years before the finding was confirmed in a randomized clinical trial.[23]

Details on tea, coffee, and alcohol consumption were routinely recorded and, although these substances might not be truly regarded as drugs, the data were studied in detail to see if there might be any unsuspected associations between their use and various clinical conditions. In this way it was noted that regular coffee drinking was associated with non-fatal myocardial infarction and that there appeared to be a dose-response relationship.[24] Heavy coffee drinkers were found to be at approximately twice the risk of being admitted to hospital with a myocardial infarction, but the risk was found to be independent of age, sex, and various risk factors for ischemic heart disease.

Studies of this type on pre-hospital drug use (with the exception of tea, coffee, and alcohol) would nowadays be best addressed using a record linkage system, but such systems were not available during the period when BCDSP was gathering in-patient data at its peak. The system that they used, in spite of the difficulties with recall bias, undoubtedly provided much valuable and hitherto unpublished information.

OTHER INTENSIVE HOSPITAL-BASED COHORT STUDIES

Routine monitoring of medical patients was carried out in Switzerland after 1974 in a program called Comprehensive Hospital Drug Monitoring - Berne (C.H.D.M.B.). This program gathered data on more that 17,000 medical patients and produced findings on a wide variety of topics.[25,26] The size of their database was comparable to that of the Boston group and many of their findings confirmed those in Boston although certain discrepancies were noted.

Children have been monitored, most successfully by Mitchell and colleagues.[27] BCDSP began to monitor children but stopped because reaction rates were very low and they felt that little useful information could be gained. Mitchell has used a similar technique and has successfully monitored large numbers of patients.

Surgical patients have been monitored by BCDSP although the number was modest. A general review of this information showed, not surprisingly, that these patients were exposed to larger numbers of drugs than medical patients and also detected a significant number of ADR.[28] These surgical data have been used for more detailed descriptive study, for example, in work that assessed the frequency of respiratory events occurring after general anaesthesia.[29]

ADVANTAGES AND DISADVANTAGES OF THE INTENSIVE HOSPITAL-BASED METHOD

The system of intensive inpatient monitoring has been shown to be extremely successful in the general hospital setting. The main strength has been the very broad comprehensive nature of the surveillance of short term in-hospital drug use. The inclusion of information on demography and social habits has broadened the scope of the program. The expansion of the system to run in different hospitals in different countries has allowed various comparisons to be made, not only in ADR incidence but also in drug utilization. The cohort approach is most likely to yield useful results in situations where drugs may cause significant increases in already high baseline risks of events or illnesses. Examples of these are noted in the preceding paragraphs.

There are many disadvantages in using the intensive hospital-based approach. Chronic drug use in the community over the period before the hospitalization cannot be assessed in any detail. The use of monitors is labor intensive and the entire approach is, therefore, expensive, particularly when compared with newer computer-based approaches such as record linkage. In contrast to the general hospital environment, where the method works well because of relatively standardized patient presentation, investigation, treatment, and prescribing, this approach is not suitable for use in many specialist units such as intensive care. In such a setting, drug use is a complicated and rapidly changing clinical feature and, even if the information could be recorded accurately by a monitor, it would be extremely complex and almost impossible to analyze successfully. Any attempt to attribute causality in such a situation, where extremely ill patients are treated with such complex drug regimes, would be impossible. The technique is unlikely to be useful in the post-marketing surveillance of new chemical entities. Such drugs will usually take some time to reach significant levels of usage in hospital, so there may be a significant time lag before a clinically significant ADR could be detected using the hospital-based approach. Occasional case reports of ADRs to a new drug might be reported, but the spontaneous reporting systems are better equipped to deal with that aspect of surveillance.

Future Uses of the Intensive Hospital-Based Approach

The main reason why regulators, the pharmaceutical industry, and the academic community should retain an interest in this rather old-fashioned approach, is that the main body of information gathered is now about fifteen years old. The period 1966 to

1975 was comprehensively covered and much new and previously unsuspected information emerged from that body of information. Since then, however, there have been a number of spectacular occurrences of ADRs occurring with new drugs such as practolol[30,31] and benoxaprofen.[32] In addition to such cases where definite problems have been discovered, various entire new categories of drugs have come into use, such as angiotensin converting enzyme inhibitors, histamine receptor antagonists, and calcium channel blockers, not to mention innumerable new individual drugs from commonly used classes such as antibiotics and beta blockers. Adverse effects of these drugs may well exist and comprehensive monitoring as described here may be of considerable benefit. In addition to the problem of new drugs, there is the distinct possibility that, after a period of time, new patterns of ADRs could emerge with the continued use of established drugs. Such drugs may find new indications for use, so entire new groups of patients might become exposed and hence be at risk of adverse effects. Established drugs may find a resurgence of use, possibly in new formulations. A good example of this was the use of slow release indomethacin in the proprietary preparation Osmosin.[33] Political and economic pressures may come to bear on patterns of hospitalization so the hospitalized population of today might be quite different from that of fifteen years ago, consequently their drug use patterns may be quite different and ADR profiles may have changed significantly.

For all these reasons there is some justification for repeating this type of intensive monitoring program every ten years or so, so that information on drug therapy and on clinical practice is kept up to date.

The difficulty of gathering very little information on new drugs using the general monitoring approach can be overcome, to a certain extent, by using a targeted drug-specific approach. This is a variation of the basic method whereby, rather than selecting a hospital service and studying all patients and all drugs, a specific drug of interest is selected and all users of that drug in the hospital are studied in detail. In this system, one can see the overlap that exists with post-marketing surveillance studies. Again, the method has been used by the Boston group to study various drugs, including cimetidine.[34] In this approach the broad aims and objectives as described previously do not apply, but the resources can be focused on a particular drug of interest and information about short-term toxicity is much more likely to be acquired quickly.

Another way in which the intensive hospital-based method could be further adapted for future use, would be to focus on specific patient groups of particular interest. One such group would be elderly persons, arbitrarily defined as those aged over 65 years. This section of the population now comprises about 15% of the total population of the United Kingdom and, although that proportion may not change much over the next few years, the shift in age distribution will continue and there will be a further increase in the population fraction aged over 80 or 85 years. This elderly group consumes between two and three times their share of drugs compared with the population average and, for various reasons, the incidence of ADRs in the elderly is also disproportionately high.[35,36] Hurwitz found an increased incidence of ADRs in the over 60 age group.[37] Williamson and Chopin[38] found a high rate of ADRs in a group of admissions to geriatric assessment units and also documented the drugs most frequently responsible. There are many and varied reasons why elderly people are likely to be more susceptible to the adverse affects of drugs. These include polypharmacy, altered pharmacokinetics, and altered pharmacodynamics in old age. There are certain difficulties in attributing causality when considering ADRs in the elderly. These include difficulties in ascertaining drug exposure, and also difficulties in assessing outcome events, particularly in patients who suffer from many different diseases concurrently.

For all these reasons, the elderly are a group worthy of detailed study in a variety of ways, including spontaneous reporting and record linkage studies. Until now, inpatient monitoring systems for assessing ADRs in elderly subjects have been confined to acute wards, and there may well be a place for a large intensive hospital-based study of institutionalized elderly subjects, possibly in chronic care.

In the light of recent developments in the assessment of ADRs, notably the development of large multi-purpose databases and record linkage, the technique of intensive hospital-based monitoring, essentially a series of simultaneous cohort studies, is often now seen as rather old fashioned and out of date, and having little role in the gathering of new knowledge. For reasons outlined in this article, it does seem that the technique may still have a part to play, albeit a relatively small one among the various methods available for the systematic study of ADRs. It should be restricted to the study of selected drugs in specific circumstances or to the study of selected patient groups. A more general approach could be justified, but only if undertaken periodically and for a finite period.

REFERENCES

1. D. P. Barr, Hazards of modern diagnosis and therapy - the price we pay, *J Amer Med Assoc*. 159:1452 (1955).
2. W. R. Best, Chloramphenicol-associated blood dyscrasias, A review of cases submitted to the American Medical Association Registry, *JAMA*. 201:181 (1967).
3. W. Lenz, Thalidomide and congenital abnormalities, *Lancet*. 1:45 (1962).
4. D. J. Finney, The design and logic of a monitor of drug use, *J Chronic Dis*. 18;77 (1965).
5. L. G. Seidl, G. F. Thornton, J. W. Smith and et. al., Studies on the epidemiology of adverse drug reactions, III. Reactions in patients on a general medical service, *Bull Johns Hopkins Hosp*. 119:299 (1966).
6. N. Hurwitz, and O. L. Wade, Intensive hospital monitoring of adverse reactions to drugs, *Br Med J*. 1;531 (1969).
7. D. Slone, H. Jick, I. Borda and et. al., Drug surveillance utilizing nurse monitors, *Lancet*. 2:901 (1966).
8. H. Jick, O. S. Miettinen, S. Shapiro and et. al., Comprehensive drug surveillance, *JAMA*. 213:1455 (1970).
9. D. H. Lawson, and H. Jick, Drug prescribing in hospitals: an international comparison, *Am J Public Health*. 66:644 (1977).
10. D. H. Lawson, Intravenous fluids in medical inpatients, *Br J Clin Pharmacol*. 4:299 (1977).
11. J. Porter, and H. Jick, Drug related deaths among medical inpatients, *JAMA*. 237:289 (1977).
12. H. Jick, D. Slone, I. Borda and et. al.: Efficacy and toxicity of heparin in relation to age and sex. *N Engl J. Med*. 279:284 (1968).
13. A. M. Walker, and H. Jick, Predictors of bleeding during heparin therapy. *JAMA*. 244:1209 (1980).
14. D. H. Lawson, D. Gloss, and H. Jick, Adverse reactions to methyldopa with special reference to hypotension, *Am Heart J*. 96:572 (1978).
15. Boston Collaborative Drug Surveillance Program: Diphenylhydantoin side effects and serum albumin levels, *Clin Pharmacol Ther*. 14:529 (1973).
16. R. R. Miller, J. Porter, and D. J. Greenblatt, Clinical importance of the interaction of phenytoin and isoniazid, *Chest*. 75:356 (1979).
17. Boston Collaborative Drug Surveillance Program: Clinical depression of the central nervous system due to diazepam and chlordiazepoxide in relation to cigarette smoking and age, *N Engl J Med*. 288:277 (1973).
18. H. Jick, and J. Porter, Drug-induced gastrointestinal bleeding, *Lancet*. 2:87 (1978).
19. D. Slone, H. Jick, G. P. Lewis, et. al., Intravenously given ethacrynic acid and gastrointestinal bleeding, *JAMA*. 209:1668 (1969).
20. R. R. Miller, Hospital admissions due to adverse drug reactions, *Arch Intern Med*. 134:219 (1974).
21. Boston Collaborative Drug Surveillance Program: Regular aspirin intake and acute myocardial infarction, *Br Med J* 1:440 (1974).
22. H. Jick, and O. S. Miettinen, Regular aspirin use and myocardial infarction, *Br Med J* 1:1057 (1976).
23. Preliminary report: findings from the aspirin component of the ongoing physicians' health study, *N Engl J Med* 318:262 (1988).
24. Boston Collaborative Drug Surveillance Program: Coffee drinking and acute myocardial infarction, *Lancet*. 2:1278 (1972).
25. M. Zoppi, M. Torok, D. Stoller-Guleryaz and et. al., Adverse drug reactions as probable causes of death, Results of the Comprehensive Hospital Drug Monitoring Berne (CHDMB), *Swiss Med J*. 112:1808 (1982).

26. M. Torok, M. Zoppi, P. Winzenried and et. al., Drug related death among 17,285 inpatients in the divisions of internal medicine of two teaching hospitals in Berne 1974-1980, p. 79, *in*: "The Impact of Computer Technology on Drug Information," P. Manell, S. G. Johansson, eds., Amsterdam, North Holland (1982).

27. A. A. Mitchell, P. Goldman, S. Shapiro, and et. al., Drug utilization and reported adverse reactions in hospitalized children, *Am J Epidemiol.* 110:196 (1979).

28. Boston Collaborative Drug Surveillance Program: Drug monitoring of surgical patients, *JAMA.* 248:1482 (1982).

29. K. Beard, H. Jick, and A. M. Walker, Adverse respiratory events occurring in the recovery room after general anesthesia, *Anesthesiology.* 64:269 (1986).

30. P. Wright, Untoward effects associated with practolol administration: oculomucocutaneous syndrome, *Br Med J.* 1:595 (1975).

31. R. H. Felix, F. A. Ive, and M. S. C. Dahl, Skin reactions to beta blockers, *Br Med J.* 1:626 (1975).

32. H. M. Taggart, and J. M. Alderdice, Fatal cholestatic jaundice in elderly patients taking benoxaprofen, *Br Med J.* 284:1372 (1982).

33. T. K. Day, Intestinal perforation associated with osmotic slow release indomethacin capsules, *Br Med J.* 287:1671 (1983).

34. J. B. Porter, K. Beard, A. M. Walker and et. al., Intensive hospital monitoring study of intravenous cimetidine, *Arch Intern Med.* 146:2237 (1986).

35. E. Grundy, Mortality and morbidity among the old, *Br Med J.* 288:663 (1984).

36. Medication for the elderly, A report of the Royal College of Physicians, *J Royal College Phys London.* 18:7 (1984).

37. N. Hurwitz, Predisposing factors in adverse reaction to drugs, *Br Med J.* 1:536 (1969).

38. J. Williamson, J. M. Chopin, Adverse reactions to prescribed drugs, *Age Aging.* 9:73 (1980).

HOSPITAL-BASED ADVERSE REACTION AND DRUG UTILIZATION REVIEW

IN THE UNITED STATES

Brian L. Strom, M.D., M.P.H.

Clinical Epidemiology Unit
Section of General Internal Medicine
Department of Medicine
University of Pennsylvania School of Medicine
Philadelphia, Pennsylvania 19104-6095

Based on data from intensive hospital-based adverse drug reaction monitoring, as many as 30% of hospitalized patients may have major or minor adverse drug reactions.[1] There are 700,000,000 U.S. exposures to drugs in hospitals each year. One-quarter to one-third of all drug use in the United States is in hospitals, and 30% of new chemical entities approved by the FDA are intended primarily for hospital use. Finally, of the 51,000 adverse drug reactions received by FDA in 1988, only 1,300 were received from hospitals (personal communication from Gerald Faich, M.D., M.P.H., formally of the FDA). As such, considerable scientific information is potentially missing about the adverse effects of drugs used in hospitals. In addition, preventable adverse drug reactions represent a major issue regarding the quality of care in hospitals. For both of these reasons, the evaluation of the use and effects of drugs in hospitals is an important problem, and one which is not being addressed well. This paper will describe the experience of one particular university hospital, as an example of developments in hospital-based pharmacoepidemiology in the U.S. which are ultimately likely to have major impact worldwide.

THE SETTING

The Hospital of the University of Pennsylvania is the major academic teaching hospital for the University of Pennsylvania School of Medicine. It is the first university-based hospital in the country, and it includes 701 beds. In early 1989, the Hospital of the University of Pennsylvania underwent its routine accreditation review by the Joint Commission on Accreditation of Health Care Organizations (JCAHO). Hospitals must be accredited by the JCAHO in order to be eligible for reimbursement by Medicare. During this accreditation review, the hospital was criticized for the absence of 1) an adverse drug reaction monitoring program, and 2) a drug use evaluation program. Simultaneously, the hospital was faced with an operating deficit of $14 million for that year.

THE SOLUTION

In response, the hospital formed a new program responsible for adverse drug reaction reporting, drug usage evaluation, and pharmacy cost containment. The goals of the new program were 1) to improve the quality of patient care by improving the clinical use of medications and minimizing adverse drug reactions, 2) to decrease hospital costs by eliminating the inappropriate use of drugs or by offering acceptable low-cost substitutions, 3) to decrease legal liability associated with the inappropriate use of high risk drugs, 4) to bring the hospital into compliance with Joint Commission requirements, and 5) to contribute new methodology and new clinical information to hospital pharmacoepidemiology.

The operational plan proposed was to hire staff and purchase equipment, to create an oversight committee, to initiate the adverse drug reaction monitoring program, to initiate the cost containment program, and then to begin the evaluation component of the drug use evaluation program. The intervention component of the drug use evaluation program was to follow later, and would be followed in turn by a reevaluation, to be certain that drug use problems that were identified were successfully addressed.

The Adverse Drug Reaction program began by developing an operational definition of adverse drug reactions of interest; publicizing the program to nurses and physicians; receiving spontaneous telephone reports of adverse drug reactions; screening computerized discharge diagnoses for adverse drug reactions; targeting selected drugs, patients, sites, etc. for intensive follow-ups; triaging reports regarding their need for in depth investigation and their need for reporting to FDA; analyzing the cumulated ADR's and reporting the results to the oversight committee; and developing plans for necessary follow-up. One category of ADR's considered as high priority for this program were those that were dose-related, and thereby potentially preventable. In addition, ADR's were considered high priority if they were "FDA reportable." "FDA reportable" adverse drug reactions were defined using the criteria FDA has imposed on manufacturers.[2] In particular, we considered FDA reportable adverse drug reactions to be those that were unlabelled, adverse reactions to drugs marketed within the last three years, and those that were serious. By "serious adverse drug reactions" we meant drug reactions which prolonged or caused hospitalization, resulted in or contributed to death, were life-threatening, or resulted in persistent or significant disability, including all cancers and birth defects.

The process of the Drug Use Evaluation program was to choose drugs for initial evaluation, to develop criteria for appropriate use, to develop chart abstracting data entry forms, to identify exposed patients using the pharmacy computer, to conduct chart reviews, to analyze the data, to report the results to the oversight committee, and then to design one or more interventions as needed to address any problems identified. Initial target drugs of the Drug Use Evaluation program were expected to result from the signals we saw from our Adverse Drug Reaction monitoring program.

The Cost Containment program was designed to identify potential problem areas, based on adverse drug reaction reports, drug use evaluations, and/or drugs generating the most expense for the hospital. Our plans were to intercede to reduce costs, using educational campaigns, formulary modifications, or other interventions, as felt necessary.

INITIAL RESULTS

During the year preceding the Joint Commission accreditation visit, a total of four adverse drug reactions were reported from our hospital. After the Joint Commission visit, because of the concerns generated, we began to receive between 2 and 11 reports of adverse drug reactions each month. In September of 1989 the Drug Use and Effects Committee (DUEC) was formed, with its associated staff. Spontaneous reports of adverse reactions increased from an average of less than 10 a month to over 30 a month. Beginning February of 1990 we began weekly or biweekly contact with selected subspecialty services, seeking adverse drug reactions. This doubled our reports to over 60 a month. We also began to review computerized discharge diagnoses for adverse drug reactions. This yielded another 50 ADR's per month. Most of the latter were reasons for admission, rather than ADR's developed in the hospital, and did not overlap much with the other ADR's being received. Finally, in addition to spontaneous reports from physicians, spontaneous reports from pharmacists, and our biweekly contact with selected subspeciality services, we regularly reviewed the charts of patients who had "critical" abnormal laboratory values, abnormal drug levels, or received antidote drugs (e.g., naloxone, protamine), adding up to another 50 ADR's a month.

Included as examples of some of the ADR's we were seeing were a series of patients with life-threatening hypotension due to protamine. In response, we are performing a formal drug use evaluation of protamine as a cohort study, to quantitate the incidence of such adverse effects, which is not now known. In addition, we will perform a case-control study comparing those who suffered these reactions to those who did not, trying to identify risk factors for them.

We also identified series of patients with lymphoreticular malignancies from OKT3, a new drug used for transplantation. In response to this, we hope to perform a nationwide case-control study, perhaps funded by the manufacturer of the drug, comparing transplant patients with lymphoreticular malignancies to those without them, exploring whether OKT3 is an unique problem here and, if so, whether there is any special population at risk. As another example, we sought to replace our cephalosporin with an NMTT-side chain containing cephalosporin, as the latter was much less expensive. However, it is uncertain whether the latter results in an increased risk of bleeding. We have just been funded by one manufacturer to perform a cohort study exploring this question. As another example we have observed a patient who suffered such severe liver disease from diclofenac that they need to undergo liver transplantation. The transplant had to be repeated and, ultimately, the patient died. Finally, we are seeing a considerable number of iatrogenic overdoeses of theophylline, digoxin, phenytoin, etc., and these are other subjects of our first drug use evaluations.

In summary, this new program is already showing signs of providing much clinically useful information. Because of Joint Commission requirements, it is likely to be duplicated in some form in every hospital in the United States. As such, the field of pharmacoepidemiology is likely to be seeing considerable new information emerging from US hospitals in the future.

REFERENCES

1.   H. Jick, Drugs - remarkably nontoxic, *New Engl J Med.* 291:824-8 (1974).
2.   C. Baum and C. Anello, The spontaneous reporting system in the United States, *in*: "Pharmacoepidemiology," B. L. Strom, ed., Churchill Livingstone, New York, 107-118 (1989).

APPROACHES TO EVALUATING CAUSATION OF

SUSPECTED DRUG REACTIONS

Judith K. Jones M.D., Ph.D.

Georgetown University
and The Degge Group, Ltd.
Washington, D.C.

THE CONTEXT OF DETERMINING CAUSALITY IN OVERALL RISK ASSESSMENT

Knowledge about an adverse drug effect typically starts out as a signal of a possible problem, usually identified through spontaneous reports of a suspected adverse drug reaction. As diagrammed in Figure 1, this signal is verified in an iterative fashion, either through further reports or studies of its biological plausibility and, if important, it is quantitated with epidemiological or, rarely, experimental studies (clinical trials). Although often taken for granted, the driving force for this iteration is often based on the

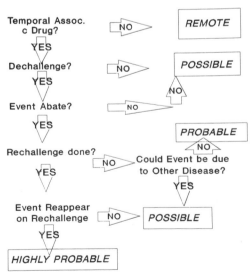

Figure 1.   The "FDA" Algorithm used in the early 1980's as a management tool for evaluating the spontaneous reports received. This was not used to actually label an event "causally related," but rather to identify those cases which were well documented (e.g., those probable or highly probable).

Drug Epidemiology and Post-Marketing Surveillance, Edited by B.L. Strom and G. Velo, Plenum Press, New York, 1992

assumption or determination, through some means, that there is a cause-effect relationship between the purported risk and the pharmaceutical. This *qualitative* part of risk assessment which evaluates a signal is an important initial part of the process.

To consider this process in detail, the *clinical event*, associated with a number of factors (drugs, diseases, diet, genetics, environment) which might cause it, can be expressed at several levels. First, it can be detected as an *Event*, in which case it is recorded (in the medical record, the medical financial receipt), and is thus available for epidemiological study.

At the next level, this event might be *attributed* to a drug. This is usually, but not always, a "global judgment"[1] of a causal association. In an epidemiologic study, it might be specifically noted as an adverse reaction in a hospital chart, or a medical bill for financial reimbursement with a code denoting drug association.

Finally, rather uncommonly, the *event*, attributed to a drug, might actually be reported to a regulatory agency or pharmaceutical company as a suspected adverse reaction, a process often accompanied by additional implications of a causal association, and often taking into account a temporal relationship, lack of confounding factors, and supportive data on dechallenge and/or rechallenge.

In theory, an event is either caused (wholly or partially) by a drug (probability = 1.0), or *not caused* by this drug (probability of 0.0). In reality, an *event* is ensconced within a milieu of not only this drug, but other possible causes, including other drugs and diseases. Practically, a judgment of probability of association <1.0 but > 0.0 will be made, for there will always be degrees of uncertainty about the association, or the lack thereof. The different ways in which this real world probability is estimated, both in the past and more recently, is the subject of this paper.

The goals of this paper are to briefly describe the emergence of causality concepts in both epidemiology and in the drug field, the evolution of progressively more structured methods requiring more information, into the present development of the Bayesian probability assessment which requires more information within a more flexible structure. These methods will then be critiqued and the uses of causality in pharmacoepidemiology and drug evaluation will be considered. Finally, some important concepts for future consideration are introduced, to improve information gathering and inference about drug risk and benefit.

DEVELOPMENT OF CONCEPTS OF CAUSALITY

Although the convergence of epidemiology and drug risk research is relatively recent, it is interesting to compare the parallel development of notions of causality in both fields.

In epidemiology, Yerushalmy and Parker[1] adapted from the original Koch-Henle postulates (used in infectious disease) five general criteria for a causal association within chronic epidemiology studies. Although argued at the time, these criteria are generally accepted:

1.   The *consistency* of an association.
2.   The *strength* of an association.
3.   The *specificity* of an association.
4.   The appropriate *temporal relationship* of an association;
5.   The *biological plausibility* of an association.

Not long thereafter, both Nelson Irey[2], researching the pathology of drug-associated disorders, and the clinical pharmacologists Karch and Lasagna[3], frustrated with the vagaries of global clinical judgment, developed structured methods for the evaluation of suspected adverse reactions, to improve inter-rater reliability. Both methods contained requirements for:

1.   Evidence of *prior experience*, analogous to the consistency requirement;
2.   The effect of *dechallenge and rechallenge* relative to disappearance and reappearance, respectively, of a suspected event, implicitly testing the strength of the association in character and time.

3. Consideration of *confounding* or other causal factors, roughly similar to a converse specificity criterion; and
4. A *temporal* relationship.

Practically, however, these drug reaction causality criteria differed from the epidemiology criteria to some extent, as shown in Table 1, based on the differing nature of data and studies relating to the consideration of causality. With progressive application of epidemiological methods to questions of adverse drug adverse reactions, appreciation of both views is relevant to the analysis of data from both spontaneous report and epidemiological sources.

TYPES OF CAUSALITY ASSESSMENTS

The methods of causality assessment can be classified in four general groups, summarized in Table 2. The first method, actually a default, or lack of a method, is *clinical judgment*, or, as described by Lane and Hutchinson, "global introspection."[4] This refers to an ill-defined process of making clinical attribution which is based on the clinical experience and individual knowledge based on the individual making the judgment. The steps for arriving at the judgment are usually not applied in any ordered way. This approach is the most commonly used in a wide variety of settings, ranging from the bedside, where the busy clinician makes a clinical assessment based on a wide variety of factors in no particular order, to regulatory agencies, who request judgements from experts, who likewise use their scientific and clinical experience to judge a particular event. As forcefully argued by Lane and Hutchinson, such judgements are fraught with inconsistencies and inter-rater scores are typically low, as was also discovered by Karch and Lasagna.

The next approach is embodied in several methods *(Algorithms with Verbal judgements)* which propose various logical structured approaches to the assessment. These typically use a flow chart or sequential assessment (algorithm), which has the effect of consistently describing the amount of information which does or does not support a causal association. Following the Irey and Karch & Lasagna approaches, they all consider timing, dechallenge, rechallenge, concomitant disease, and existing

Table 1.   Criteria for Causality: A Comparison of Epidemiological and Early Drug Event Causality Approaches

CRITERION	EPIDEMIOLOGY	ADR CAUSALITY
Data	Populations	Single Clinical Cases
Consistency	Repeated findings in multiple studies	Repeated reports
Specificity	Specificity of association in studies	Lack of other causes
Strength	Degree of association in studies	Association with dechallenge and rechallenge
Temporal Association	Temporal association established in study	Required but criteria for meeting not always clear
Biological Plausibility	Variably demonstrated	Variable-often not known

Table 2.   Types of Causality Assessment Methods

Global/Clinical Judgment

Algorithm: Verbal Judgment

Algorithm with Numerical Scoring

Probabilistic

---

knowledge. The FDA algorithm, developed and used until the late 1980's, is an example of this (Figure 1).[5] It was purposely devised to be simple, to allow its use for variably trained professionals. Because the FDA was often the first recipient of a new effect, the criterion for previous knowledge of the reaction was omitted. It is important to note that this algorithm was not used for true causality judgements; rather, it was a management tool to identify the more well-documented suspect cases (usually probably or highly probably associated).

With the recognition that verbal conclusions of "possible" and "probable" were ambiguous, new methods (*Algorithms with Numerical Scoring of Individual Judgments*) were spawned that provided for scoring of answers to the basic questions of previous knowledge, timing, etc., as in Kramer, Hutchinson, et al's elaborate algorithm.[6] In some cases, as in the extensive Venulet algorithm[7] and the Naranjo algorithm,[8] additional *types* of questions appeared. The French algorithm,[9] embodied within France's drug regulatory requirements, can be classified in this group. An example of this type, used by many hospitals and manufacturers, the Naranjo approach is summarized in Table 3.

It is apparent from this and the other more elaborate methods, that they represent efforts to identify more criteria to address the low specificity of the earlier methods. These additional criteria related to the *history* of the patient's experience with the drug or similar drugs, and the *character of the event*. Questions relating to the standard criteria were also expanded. Thus, the approach to the causality problem increasingly required a more detailed look at the event. This evolution in thinking set the stage for the next approach, which is based on a very detailed examination of *both* the prior evidence, as well as the specific details of the case, to determine the *probability* of drug causation.

Three conferences probably provided the setting for this progression of thinking. The first, held at Morges, Switzerland in 1983 and summarized in a published monograph,[10] was a gathering of many of those who had originally developed the methods. The goal was an exchange of information and the first attempt to identify whether there was any basis for a "standard" method. The second, held in 1984 in Crystal City, Virginia, again brought together the algorithm developers and carried out specific comparisons using standard cases.[11] However, in an effort to get a fresh look at the topic, a theoretical statistician, Dr. David Lane, was invited to critique to proceedings and suggest new approaches. His critique[4] marked one of the beginnings of the development of the Bayesian probabilistic approach to causality. The other complementary one was in France, where there was considerable interest in causality and where Auriche had also proposed a probabilistic approach. The third meeting, held in Paris shortly after the second, included most of the participants at the second, and following this a group was formed to develop and apply the proposed Bayesian method to the causality assessment of adverse reactions.[12] Since that time, a number of articles have demonstrated its application and a specific conference was held to demonstrate its use.[13,14] More recently, two of the members of the original working group (Naranjo and Hutchinson) have developed automated versions of the method.[15]

The *Bayesian approach* to evaluating a suspected adverse event evaluates the posterior probability, or odds, of an event, given causation by the suspected drug, versus

Table 3.   The Naranjo Algorithm and Types of Data Requiring Judgments

| QUESTION | ANSWER SCORE | | | TYPE OF CRITERION |
	Yes	No	UNK	
1. Previous *conclusive* reports of reaction?	+1	0	0	PRIOR EVIDENCE
2. Did event appear after drug given?	+2	-1	0	TEMPORAL
3. Did event abate after drug removed *or* specific antagonist given?	+1	0	0	DECHALLENGE
4. Did reaction reappear when drug re-administered?	+2	-1	0	RECHALLENGE
5. Are there alternative causes which could have caused event?	-1	+2	0	CONFOUNDERS
6. Did reaction reappear when placebo given?	-1	+1	0	RECHALLENGE
7. Was drug detected in blood at toxic levels?	+1	0	0	CHARACTER
8. Was reaction dose-related?	+1	0	0	CHARACTER
9. Past history of similar event with similar or same drug?	+1	0	0	PRIOR HISTORY
10. Was event confirmed by objective evidence?	+1	0	0	CHARACTER
TOTAL SCORE				

the probability of the event, given non-(suspect)drug causation. This involves considering: (1) the prior probability of the event being associated with the drug versus non-drug, and (2) the probabilities associated with *each component* of the suspected reaction, termed the likelihood ratios, as expressed in the equation in Figure 2. The prior information can often be derived from clinical trial and epidemiological studies, if available. The likelihood ratios are determined from a detailed examination of the case over a time line as illustrated in Figure 3, and the example in Figure 4 indicating the sequential analysis of each component of the likelihood ratio. This method requires a much more rigorous analysis. First, the event must be defined relatively precisely. Second, the time period in which the appearance of the event must be selected, based on the event type and case. Then, *all information* available must be used to evaluate both the

Prior and Likelihood ratios for both drug and non-drug causation. This ideally requires an extensive literature search.[13,14] The resulting *Estimate of Posterior Probability* is a time-dated estimate. This is because the evaluation typically identifies, via a sensitivity analysis, the pivotal data which determines the estimate, and in some cases this can be investigated and clarified. To date, this approach has pointed out the limited state of information about not only drug-associated disease, but also about the actual characteristics of most clinical events with respect to their timing, character, etc.

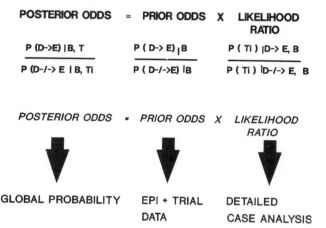

BAYESIAN APPROACH

$$\textbf{POSTERIOR ODDS} = \textbf{PRIOR ODDS} \times \textbf{LIKELIHOOD RATIO}$$

$$\frac{P(D{\to}E)|B, T}{P(D{\text{-}/\text{-}}E\,|\,B,\,Ti)} \qquad \frac{P(D{\to}E)|B}{P(D{\text{-}/{\to}}E)|B} \qquad \frac{P(Ti)|D{\text{-}}E,\,B}{P(Ti)|D{\text{-}/\text{-}}E,\,B}$$

$$POSTERIOR\ ODDS = PRIOR\ ODDS \times LIKELIHOOD\ RATIO$$

GLOBAL PROBABILITY   EPI + TRIAL DATA   DETAILED CASE ANALYSIS

Figure 2.   Equation for the Bayesian Analysis of Suspected Adverse Reactions based on Bayes theorem.

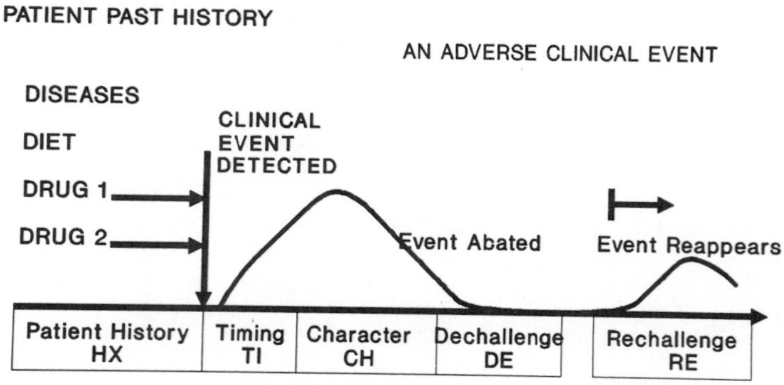

PATIENT PAST HISTORY

AN ADVERSE CLINICAL EVENT

DISEASES

DIET   CLINICAL EVENT DETECTED

DRUG 1

DRUG 2   Event Abated   Event Reappears

Patient History HX	Timing TI	Character CH	Dechallenge DE	Rechallenge RE

Figure 3.   The Time Line of a Case or suspected drug-associated event, used as the basis for Likelihood Ratio analysis.

BAYESIAN APPROACH

POSTERIOR ODDS = PRIOR ODDS X   P (C) | Given D -> E, B

LR = LIKELIHOOD RATIO   ————————————————

= LR =   X LR =   X LR =   P (C) | Given D -/->E, B
  (History) (Timing) (Characteristics)

    X LR =   X LR =
    (Dechallenge) (Rechallenge = 1)   etc.

EXAMPLE

$$\mathrm{LR}_{(Dechal)} = \frac{P\ (Dechallenge\ +)\ |\ Given\ D\text{->}E,\ \&\ B,\ History,\ Timing,\ Char.}{P\ (Dechallenge\ +)\ |\ Given\ D/\text{->}E,\ B,\ History,\ Timing,\ Char.}$$

Figure 4.   The overall likelihood ratio broken down into components for calculation of individual components related to a chronological analysis of the case.

A very simple case is illustrated in Figure 5, which spells out the approach in a cause of suspected analgesic-associated nausea. If the information about the nausea associated with the underlying condition revealed that the probability of nausea was greatest within the first 6 hours, rather than the 48 hours, a different lower result would ensue.

This approach to a causality assessment has been both praised as the "gold standard" of methods and criticized as far too complex for practical use.[13] Nonetheless, it has primarily been promoted as an approach most important when the first serious reaction is reported, if this is pivotal for a decision about either the continued development of a drug (in the Phase II or III clinical trial period) or the continued marketing of a drug (in Phase IV). It offers the most rigorous, structured approach to understanding the relationship, if any, between the event and the suspected drug. The result of such an analysis not only provides an estimate of probable association, but also a "map" of research questions to be addressed if further research is done and a case definition for further epidemiological research. Further, the usefulness of the method will be considerably enhanced with the advent of the automated methods, such as MacBARDI.[15]

USES OF THE METHODS

Examination of the use, or lack of use, of these methods is revealing. In France, the French method has become a part of the regulatory requirements, so that each event reported to either a center for pharmacovigilance or a manufacturer is subjected to a standardized method. Royer, head of the French Pharmacovigilance committee has noted that, at the very least, the use of this approach has facilitated the collection of standard data on suspected reactions, which, in turn, helps in interpretation.[17] The use of structured causality methods by other regulatory agencies varies, but primarily uses relatively simple methods with verbal, rather than numerical, methods.

The pharmaceutical industry is divided in its use of causality methods. In the U.S., relatively few manufacturers use a formal method, partially out of concern for the legal and regulatory implications. Abroad, usage varies and may even be applied either in some areas (e.g., postmarketing drug safety) and not others and informally, or for research purposes only, but use is not widely publicized at the present.

Nonetheless, based on discussions of causality, in meetings and in such forums as the newsletter of the international organization devoted to the examination of adverse reaction causality-the Associated Permanent Workshop of Imputologists[18], uses of the methods are either for practical and/or scientific purposes.

BAYESIAN APPROACH

POSTERIOR ODDS = PRIOR ODDS x LIKELIHOOD RATIO

EXAMPLE (After Lane, et al: P'ceut. Med. 1987:2: 265)

IF DRUG D IS ANALGESIC: CAUSES NAUSEA IN 1/8 ,
ALWAYS IN FIRST HOUR
UNDERLYING MEDICAL CONDITION M HAS NAUSEA s D IN 1/10,
ANY TIME IN FIRST TWO DAYS

EVENT = NAUSEA   TIME "HORIZON" = 2 DAYS

CASE: Pt c M, takes Drug, D, has Event (Nausea) in 45 Min.

Since History, Character = 1.0 for Drug vs. Non-Drug Nausea
and Dechallenge, Rechallenge information not present
Analysis is of Timing alone

PRIOR ODDS

P (D-> E) |B Incidence of M-caused Nausea same +/- Drug

∴ 1/8 -1/10 = 5/40-4/40 = 1/40 Due to Drug

P (D-/->E) |B 1/10 = 4/40 due to M

Of those with Nausea: $\dfrac{1/5 \text{ assoc. c Drug}}{4/5 \text{ Assoc c M}}$ = 0.25

For LR $_{(Ti)}$ P (Ti |D-> E, B) = 1.0 [All in First Hour]   1/1/48 = 48

P (Ti) |M-> E, B = 1/48 [Any time in 48 Hours]

Posterior Odds = 0.25 x 48 = 12

P (D-> E B, Ti = P/P+1 = 12/13 = 0.92

Figure 5.   A simple case analyzed by the Bayesian method. Most of the components of the likelihood ratio (history, character) are not different for drug caused and non-drug caused and are therefore = 1.0. Thus, timing is the critical data element. Analysis of the relative contribution of each component of the Posterior Odds result allows identification of the most important factors which determine the result, and by corollary, those questions which have the greatest need for research and/or verification.

The "practical" uses include:

1.   Identification of "good" cases which provide adequate data for follow-up;
2.   Identification of which cases to use for decision-making:
   a.   For labeling changes
   b.   For decisions regarding stopping a clinical trial, or even development of a drug.

Other uses of the methods include:

1.   Categorizing cases according to various attributes, which are also part of the causality assessment process, e.g., positive rechallenge cases;

2. Identifying what data is unknown and possibly critical to know about an event. For example, the timing of onset, and the presence or absence of eosinophilia associated with a drug-associated hepatic event. The sensitivity analysis portion of the Bayesian method is particularly useful for this.

SUMMARY AND FINAL REFLECTIONS

The past decade has seen the evolution of thinking about evaluation of spontaneous reports of suspected adverse reactions and adverse events in clinical trials. This evolution has built upon the basic criteria used in the early elements and has simply increased and structured the type of information used, as illustrated in Figure 6. When detailed examination is desired, an array of methods are available which can provide both some basis for structured decision-making, and for defining directions for research.

However, there is clear disagreement about the role of structured causality assessment in drug development and postmarketing safety assessment. Those with access to large numbers of reports (e.g., the large drug regulatory bodies, such as the U.S. FDA) have more recently argued that such methods are of little use and have opted for epidemiological approaches. France's approach is an important exception. Pharmaceutical manufacturers with drugs in development have, until recently, done global assessment, but little formal, causality evaluation of those critical adverse events which become pivotal for continuing the testing of a drug in clinical trials. However,

EVOLUTION OF CRITERIA, INFORMATION & JUDGEMENTS

CRITERIA/DATA	METHODS		
	VERBAL	SCORING	PROBABILITY
Prior Data on Event			
- Any	+/-	+	+
● Specific	0	0	+
Temporal			
- Event p Drug (only)	+	+	+
● Event in Appropriate Time p Drug	0	0	+
Dechallenge			
- Any Improvement	+	+	+
- Improvement c Removal	0	+	+
● Time Course Consistent	0	0	+
Rechallenge			
- Any	+	+	+
- Any +/- + Placebo Resp.	0	+	+
● Timing of Rechallenge	0	0	+
Character of Event			
- Clinical Character + Laboratory	0	+	+
● Time Course of Event	0	0	+
History of Patient			
- Other Diseases	+	+	+
- Past History Prev. Reactions		+	+
● Details of Past Hx	0	0	+

Figure 6. Evolution of Analysis of Causality of Suspected Adverse Reactions: from simple verbal algorithms to Bayesian Analysis and increase in the amount and types of information required.

several are now recognizing the value of formal methods, such as the Bayesian approach, to assist in this difficult decision-making.[16] It is fair to say that the "jury is still out" with respect to the role of structured causality assessment. It is the bias of this author that ultimately, as we increase our understanding of drug safety assessment, both premarketing and post, that causality methods will play an increasingly important role. Some of the bases for this opinion are summarized as follows:

1. If causality assessment were called "differential diagnosis," the concept would be more palatable to many, and this notion would assist in collecting better quality spontaneous reports. The primary physician reporters, familiar with this concept, would be more inclined to weigh all the possible causal factors. Thus, use of "Differential Diagnosis" or "Causality Criteria" by the primary reporting physician closest to the event would result in more complete data, possibly less biased than what is seen in the typical "adverse reaction: reporting forms.

2. Regulators will likely continue to need some types of formal assessment of single or grouped reactions in at least some cases. Not all problems can be evaluated using epidemiological methods (cost, time, and rareness of drug exposure being important reasons). Further, a defined process:
    a. Requires better data collection;
    b. Avoids arbitrariness;
    c. Makes criteria for decision-making *explicit and open*.
    d. Can serve as a useful management tool for large numbers of reactions.

3. A Bayesian approach to event assessment, particularly when routinely automated, should serve as a valuable tool for:
    a. Critical reactions, particularly in Phase II and III drug development, and in preparation for marketing;
    b. Research in drug-induced disease, in mapping out needs for data, both descriptive and epidemiologic.

Ultimately, the divergent views of proponents of epidemiology versus those who focus on causality and spontaneous reports are likely to converge as the research in both areas reveals information of value to the other. The efforts are related, as best illustrated in the two components of the Bayesian equation which combines the prior probability, based on epidemiology, with the likelihood ratios, which are best determined with a solid understanding of the characteristics and mechanisms of drug-induced disease. The process by which they converge in the coming years will be interesting, and will almost surely contribute to the understanding, management, and/or prevention of drug-associated disorders.

REFERENCES

1. A. R. Feinstein, Clinical Biostatistics. XLVII. Scientific Standards vs. statistical associations and biologic logic in the analysis of causation, *Clin Pharmacol Ther*. 25:481 (1979).
2. N. Irey, Diagnostic problems in drug-induced diseases. p. 1., in: Drug-Induced Diseases Vol. 4, L. Meyler L, H. M. Peck (eds), Elsevier Science Publishers, Amsterdam (1972).
3. F. Karch, and L. Lasagna, Toward the operational identification of adverse drug reactions, *Clin Pharmacol Ther*. 21:247 (1977).
4. D. L. Lane, A probabilist's view of Causality Assessment, *Drug Info J*. 18:323 (1984).
5. W. M. Turner, The Food and Drug Administration algorithm, *Drug Info J*. 18:259 (1984).
6. M. S. Kramer, J. M. Levanthal, T. A. Hutchinson, and et. al., An algorithm for the operation al assessment of adverse drug reactions, I. Background, description and instructions for use, *J Am Med Assoc*. 242:623 (1979).
7. J. Venulet, A. G. Ciucci, G. C. Berneker, Updating of a method for causality assessment of adverse drug reactions, *Int J Clin Pharmacol*. 24:559 (1986).

8. C. A. Naranjo, U. Busto, E. M. Sellers, and et al, A method for estimating the probability of adverse drug reactions, *Clin Pharmacol Ther.* 30:239 (1981).

9. B. Bégaud, J. C. Evreux, J. Jouglard and et. al., Unexpected or toxic drug reaction assessment (imputation). Actualization of the method used in France, *Therapie.* 40:111, (1985).

10. J. Venulet, G. C. Bernaker, and A. G. Ciucci, eds. *Assessing Causes of Adverse Drug Reactions*, Academic Press, London (1982).

11. R. Herman, (ed), Drug Event Associations: Perspectives, Methods, and Users, Proceedings of the Drug Information Workshop, Arlington, VA, October-November 1983, *Drug Info J.* 18:1 (1984).

12. J. K. Jones, Drug-event Associations: A view of the current status. Epilogue, *Drug Info J.* 18:331 (1984).

13. J. K. Jones, and R. L. Herman, (eds), The Future of Adverse Drug Reaction Diagnosis: Computers, Clinical Judgment and the Logic of Uncertainty, Proceedings of the Drug Information Assocation Workshop, Arlington, VA, February 1986, *Drug Info J.* 20 (1986).

14. D. A. Lane, M. S. Kramer, T. A. Hutchinson, and et. al., The Causality Assessment of Adverse Drug Reactions using a Bayesian Approach, *Pharmaceutical Med.* 2:265 (1987).

15. K. L. Lanctot, and C. A. Naranjo, Using microcomputers to simplify the Bayesian Causality Assessment of Adverse Drug Reactions, *Pharmaceut Med.* 4:185 (1990).

16. C. A. Naranjo, K. L. Lanctot, and D. A. Lane, Bayesian differential diagnosis of neutropenia associated with antiarrhythmic agents, *J Clin Pharmacol.* 30:12990 (in press).

17. R. Royer, Personal communication.

18. A.P.W.I., Newsletter No. 1 (1989).

PHARMACOECONOMICS:

PRINCIPLES AND BASIC TECHNIQUES OF ECONOMIC ANALYSIS

Henry Glick, M.A.
Raynard Kington, M.D.

Section of General Internal Medicine
and Leonard Davis Institute of Health Economics
University of Pennsylvania
Philadelphia, Pennsylvania 19104-2676
        and
University of California-Los Angeles School of Medicine
Los Angeles, CA 90024

Economic analysis of health care, and of clinical medicine in particular, has attracted increasing attention in recent years. In part, this may reflect a growing perception that health care spending is reaching inordinate levels. Most people would agree with the view that investments in maintaining, promoting, or restoring health care are well spent. However, finite health care resources confront potentially limitless demands and, at some point, choices must be made. Economic analysis informs the process of making such choices, both among different health care technologies and between health care and other forms of investment and consumption.

While a part of the broad discipline of economic assessment, this field of study embodies terms and concepts particular to health care. Understanding of these principles is likely to greatly enhance readers' appreciation of the growing body of health economics data now appearing in the medical and economic press.

Traditionally, three issues have been addressed in the evaluation of pharmaceutical agents. The first deals with safety; ignoring any potential good the drug may do, is it harmful to people? "Traditional" pharmacoepidemiology studies are used to address this question. A second traditional set of questions in medical evaluation is that of efficacy; can a particular drug or technical intervention work? For example, under ideal conditions when a patient is given the correct dose, at the correct time, over an appropriate period, does a therapeutic agent have the desired effect? The third set of questions deals with effectiveness. Outside the ideal setting of a clinical trial, patients are sent home with a prescription and comply more or less well with the dosing and other instructions. The question now is, does the drug work in the real world when patients use it on a day-to-day basis according to their own perception (or modification) of instructions given to them by their physicians?

To these traditional analyses economists have now added a new area of evaluation, the question of efficiency. The essence of this new perspective is expressed in the question, "Are we getting the best outcome for the money we are spending?" For instance, are we spending the least we need to in order to secure a given degree of therapeutic effect? Alternatively, if we have a certain amount of money to spend, are we buying the greatest degree of therapeutic benefit achievable at that level of expenditure?

This question of efficiency is similar to the sort of decision making people undertake as part of daily routine. We add up benefits and add up costs; if the benefits outweigh the costs, we continue. The essential differences in economic assessments are

Drug Epidemiology and Post-Marketing Surveillance, Edited by B.L. Strom
and G. Velo, Plenum Press, New York, 1992

that particular rules govern the calculation of costs and benefits, and that assumptions are made explicit in a way not done in day-to-day decision making.

The effect of rules governing calculations is to impose a degree of consistency, although this may be more ideal than real. If the rules are always applied in the same way it is possible to look at the cost-effectiveness of treating one disease entity, then at the cost-effectiveness of treating another disease, and then to allocate funds across different diseases with reasonable confidence that the choices made offer the most cost-effective use of resources. In reality, such consistent application of rules does not occur. Different researchers use different methods which are not all comparable.

The second effect of having rules and explicit assumptions is that it is clear what costs have been included in the analysis and, just as importantly, what has been excluded. For example, in 1986, Nettelman et al.[1] studied the treatment of Chlamydia at a clinic for sexually transmitted diseases and concluded that the most cost-effective protocol would be to administer tetracycline for one week to all sexually active patients who presented. However, they also concluded that indiscriminate use of tetracycline could significantly alter the development of resistant organisms and hence considered it unlikely that the strategy of empiric therapy for all patients would be adopted. Thus, the authors concluded that, on the basis of their study, everyone should be treated empirically, but they do not believe this will happen, because their evaluation excluded the possible costs of development of resistance. By stating that this factor has been excluded, Nettelman et al. provide a most important additional perspective on their basic conclusion.

Economic assessment is about choosing between alternative uses of resources. In doing so, both the costs and outcomes of investments are considered. A basic assumption of any analysis is that there are not, and never will be, enough resources to satisfy all needs completely. Accordingly, trade-offs have to be made -- where to invest and where not to. If resources are applied in one way, the *opportunity* to employ them in any other way is lost. Hence, the basic unit of analysis is *opportunity cost*, where the cost of a resource is defined as being equal to the benefits that would accrue if that resource was used in its best alternative application.

Three basic concepts are involved in economic analysis of health care - the type of analysis that is performed, the types of costs and benefits that are included in the analysis, and the point of view from which the analysis is undertaken.[2] Appreciating the different dimensions is the key to understanding the analysis as a whole.

There are three types of analysis which may be performed: cost identification, cost-effectiveness, and cost-benefit. They are distinguished by whether or not benefits are assessed in the analysis, and how these benefits are quantified. Three types of costs and benefits may be considered: direct, indirect, and intangible. Finally, there are at least four points of view from which the analysis may be undertaken: that of the patient; that of the provider of health care; that of the payor; and that of society.

TYPES OF ANALYSES

Cost Identification Analyses

The first of the sets of parameters to consider is the type of analysis being performed. Cost identification (also referred to as cost minimization or cost-cost analysis) estimates the cost of an intervention, but does not calculate its benefits. This approach is appropriate when two options of equal efficacy are being compared. For example, given that two hypolipemic agents are equally efficacious, which is the cheapest to use?

Velez-Gil et al.[3] have performed a cost-identification analysis for herniorrhaphy. Given changes in surgical procedure, and the provision of postoperative care in patients' homes, they estimated that these changes would reduce the cost of a hernia operation by 75%. These savings were divided among personnel, drugs, and supplies; the potentially fixed cost of overhead and depreciation; and "hotel costs" in the hospital. Equal efficacy of the present and proposed system was assumed by positing no change in complication rates for the procedure.

Cost-Effectiveness Analysis

Cost-effectiveness analysis broadens the perspective to include both costs and outcomes. However, the costs and outcomes (or benefits) are not expressed in the same units. For example, the results of an analysis may be expressed as millions of dollars per year of life gained; here, costs are expressed in dollars, outcome in years of life gained or saved. The results of this type of analysis are meaningful primarily in comparison with other interventions. Comparison is essential in order to establish if the cost of the years of life saved is cheap or expensive, since this depends on what else might be bought with the money and what it would cost to buy a year of life by some other means.

The results of a cost-effectiveness analysis can be analyzed in two ways. One approach is to compare the cost-effectiveness ratios of the interventions (expressed for each program as costs divided by outcomes). The alternative approach is based on comparisons of incremental costs and incremental benefits. The incremental cost is the cost of the first program minus the cost of the second, divided by incremental benefits, for example, by the number of years of life gained from the first program minus the number of years gained from the second. The latter is the preferred method of analysis.

When two interventions are compared, there are four principal potential outcomes. Intervention A can cost the same or more and do less than intervention B (B is said to dominate A), or it can cost less and do the same or more (in which case A dominates B). In either case -- all other considerations being equal -- the less costly, more effective program should be adopted. The choice is less clear when intervention A costs less than B, but also does less, or when it costs more but does more. In these cases, the choice will depend on whether either or both of the cost-effectiveness ratios is acceptable and whether the incremental cost-effectiveness ratio favors intervention A or intervention B.

Consider an example of a cost-effectiveness analysis (otherwise known as a cost-utility analysis) involving treatment of Chlamydia by two alternative strategies.[1] The first involves a cervical culture for low-risk patients and empiric therapy for high-risk patients. The second strategy involves cervical and urethral cultures for low-risk patients and empiric therapy for high-risk patients. A scale was developed to rate how good the outcomes were -- i.e., the "utility" of the different regimens. Strategy 1 cost $29.84 and had a "utility" of 0.941, resulting in a cost per unit of utility of $31.71 (i.e., 29.84/0.941). The second strategy cost $33.02 and had a utility of 0.953. Hence, the cost per unit of utility was $34.65.

Strategy 1 has the lower cost-effectiveness ratio but is not automatically better than strategy 2 because, although it costs less, it also buys less. Is the additional benefit from strategy 2 worth the extra cost? The extra cost per additional unit of utility may be calculated thus:

$$\frac{Cost_2 - Cost_1}{Utility_2 - Utility_1} = \frac{\$33.02 - \$29.84}{0.953 - 0.941}$$

The answer is $265 for each additional unit of utility accruing from strategy 2. The decision to adopt strategy 1 or strategy 2 turns on whether one thinks it is worth paying an extra $265 to get that additional unit of utility. If, for instance, units of utility equated to extra years of life, most people would make this investment very readily. If a unit of utility equated to a few extra seconds of life, very few would be interested in spending the money. As this example illustrates, decisions such as these can only be made if there is some idea of how much a unit of utility is worth.

Outcomes may be described not only in terms of cost per year of life saved, but also as cost per quality-adjusted year of life (QALY) saved. The reasoning behind the concept of the QALY is that not every year gained is of equal value. For instance, saving someone who then lives on in a vegetative state is not the same as restoring a patient to full health. In recent years, economists have been moving to the QALY as the preferred basis for cost-effectiveness analysis. Costs per QALY can vary considerably. Thus, bypass grafting for left main coronary artery disease cost $4,200 per QALY saved (in 1983), whereas school tuberculosis testing programs cost as much as $43,700 per QALY gained.[4]

Why is there such a large variation in cost between the relatively sophisticated procedure of bypass grafting and the simpler process of tuberculosis testing? Bypass surgery is an intervention for an acute clinical condition. Resource expenditure is thus closely targeted to the appropriate condition and the benefits are realized more or less immediately. By contrast, the vast majority of children screened for tuberculosis will never develop the disease; those who do, often will not suffer its consequences until some point in the future. Hence, the resources available to tackle this problem are widely diffused. Moreover there is a commitment to spend resources now in order to realize gains at some point in the future. Hence, the amount of money spent for every prevented case of tuberculosis is very great.

Although the QALY has become established as a favored index of cost-effectiveness analysis, there are many other ways of expressing outcome. These include the cost per year of life gained and the cost per life saved. However, it is not always possible to quantify how medical interventions affect years of life, or lives saved. Sometimes it is impossible to report more than costs for successful treatment, or costs for cases of illness avoided. On occasion, it is not even possible to go that far. For example, in diabetes, changes in certain intermediate biochemical parameters such as fasting blood glucose can be monitored, but there is little understanding of how these relate to the course of the disease in the long term. In such cases, parameters such as cost for a percentage change in fasting blood glucose may be quoted.

Cost-Benefit Analysis

In cost-benefit analysis, costs and outcomes are considered and both factors are reported in monetary terms. If subtracting costs from benefits results in a positive value, money has been saved or benefits added; if the value is negative, money has been lost. Hence, unlike cost-effectiveness results, which are interpreted in relation to corresponding data from other programs, cost-benefit results are meaningful in themselves.

Although translating benefits into monetary terms can be extremely informative, many people find it distasteful, because it often involves putting a value on additional years of peoples' lives. This discomfort is probably one reason why cost-benefit analysis is infrequently encountered in health economic analysis.

As with cost-effectiveness analysis, there are two ways to report the results of cost-benefit analysis. One is the net benefit approach, in which the total cost is subtracted from the total benefit, both being expressed in cash terms. The second approach, now outmoded but still sometimes encountered in the literature, is the cost-benefit ratio. In this, total costs make up the numerator and total benefits constitute the denominator, the result being expressed as a ratio. The problem with the latter approach is that benefits can expressed as negative costs and costs as negative benefits. Hence, it is possible to alter the ratio by subtracting something from the numerator and moving it to the denominator or vice versa. Such changes do not affect the results of a net benefit analysis. For this reason, net benefit is the preferred technique.

Eisenberg and Kitz[5] performed a cost-benefit analysis of the cost of treating osteomyelitis in an inpatient setting, compared with a program of early discharge plus domiciliary antibiotic treatment. Costs of conventional hospital care were calculated at $2,105. For the early discharge program, the figure was $1,063. Total direct outpatient medical costs in the conventional setting were zero, but amounted to $746 for the early discharge scheme. There were savings in non-medical direct costs and in indirect costs with the early discharge program. In all, early discharge was shown to yield savings of just over $500.

TYPES OF COSTS

The second dimension of economic analysis is concerned with the types of costs and benefits that can be included in an analysis. Costs can be classified as direct, indirect or intangible. Intangible costs are hard to measure and generally involve pain and suffering, factors that are difficult to include in quantitative analyses.

Direct costs can be broken down into medical costs and non-medical costs. Direct medical costs are the medical resources consumed by the intervention --

hospitalization, physicians, pharmaceuticals, laboratory tests, and the like. Direct non-medical costs are incurred as a consequence of the treatment, for example, expenses associated with regular outpatient visits, special diets, and the installation at home of equipment or facilities to help overcome the consequences of disability. Direct costs may be fixed or variable. Fixed costs are constant and independent of the volume of services provided; variable costs fluctuate. This fluctuation may take the form of a linear increase in costs as the volume of services rises, but other patterns are possible.

X-ray facilities provide an example of the nature of fixed and variable costs. If the machine is already in place, the capital expenditure required to buy it is a fixed cost -- the price of the machine does not vary depending on its use. On the other hand, each x-ray generates a photographic plate, and the more x-rays taken, the more film is used. Film therefore constitutes a variable cost, determined by the volume of service provided. Eventually, the number of x-rays required may exceed the capacity of the machine. At that point, a new or extra machine will have to be bought. Since this is a direct consequence of the increased volume of service provided, this capital outlay qualifies as a variable cost.

Closely related to the idea of fixed and variable costs is the very important concept of marginal costs. These are the costs incurred by providing additional units of service, or the costs saved by providing fewer units of service. Marginal costs are the costs used in economic assessment of health care. Technically, marginal costs are defined as the rate of change of slope of the line describing the relation between total costs and volume of service. (Hence, marginal costs are not affected by fixed costs.) The smaller the rate of change, the smaller the marginal cost (or the smaller the marginal saving); the larger the rate of change, the larger the cost or saving. Implicit in this statement is the fact that marginal costs may vary depending on the point on the curve at which the program is evaluated.

In more practical terms, the concept of marginal cost may be understood in terms of drug costs per dose. Assume that the cost of preparing 10 doses of a given drug is $50. The average cost of a single dose is $5. When deciding whether or not to cut back to nine doses, or to prepare an eleventh dose of this drug, is the average cost per dose the appropriate figure to look at? Suppose there are substantial start-up costs associated with the manufacturing process -- substantial set-up costs, quality control, etc. -- such that it costs $49 to make nine doses of the drug, and $50 to make 10 doses. In this case, the marginal cost of providing the tenth dose is just $1. When considering whether to provide that dose, the marginal cost of $1 obviously is far more relevant than the average cost of $5.

Marginal costing is an essential principle in economic assessment of health care schemes -- what we are really interested in are the changes in costs when additional units of service are provided. Average cost is of less interest, and arguably of less value, than marginal cost. It is the latter which should be used in program evaluations. The fact that marginal cost does not equal average cost poses special problems in health care evaluation.

The standard economic assumption is that purchase price equals cost -- to find out how much something costs, it is necessary only to find out its purchase price. This is rarely the case in health care. There are a number of reasons for this disparity, which apply in different degrees in different countries.

First, there is the influence of subsidization and free care. In countries where some or all of the costs of care are met from central funds, the monetary cost of the services provided is generally not reflected in the purchase price to the beneficiary. The same is true under payment systems based on average costs, rather than the actual cost of treating a specific patient.

Health insurance also can affect the relation between cost and purchase price. An assumption in the purchase price-equals-cost model is that the people getting a service also pay for it. In these circumstances they may be expected to trade off how much they want a service against its purchase price. This ceases to be the case when costs are borne by insurance companies, with the result that patients' demand for health care is circumscribed only by their out-of-pocket and time costs.

On a more theoretical level, the price-equals-cost model requires that consumers have enough information to judge the value of what they are buying. In health care, this is often not the case. For instance, doctors usually decide if someone needs to enter hospital and how long they need to stay there. Most patients are not in a position to judge such issues, further distorting the usual economic assumptions about the relationship between price and cost.

Because of this dysjunction between price and cost in health care, special techniques have been developed to estimate costs. One such technique is called component enumeration.[6,7,8] The essence of this procedure is a detailed enumeration of all the steps involved in a process, multiplied by the wages of the people involved, plus any increments for supply costs. Summing all these factors together should establish how much it costs to provide that particular service. Other mechanisms of cost estimation rely on analysis of fees for private health care, on accounting data[9,10] (including step-down accounting techniques), and on statistical techniques such as multiple regression analysis of hospital budgets.[11]

In health care analyses the term indirect costs does not embrace the conventional accounting notion of these costs (which would include such things as electricity and water). It refers instead to the costs of morbidity and mortality. Two methods have been used to assess these costs: one is the human capital approach; the other is the willingness-to-pay approach.

The human capital approach uses lost wages or lost livelihood as a measure of the lost opportunities attributable to death and/or disability. Effectively (if perhaps pejoratively), this method equates the value of a person's life with the value of their livelihood. Willingness to pay, in essence, poses the question "How much are you willing to pay to avoid the risk of disease and/or death?"

The human capital approach - which is the method most often used to assess indirect costs - has two advantages over the willingness to pay approach. The first is that it is relatively easy to compute. Governments publish statistics on average earnings by age and sex, making it comparatively easy to calculate someone's likely loss of earnings if, for example, myocardial infarction prompts retirement 10 years ahead of expectation. In addition, this technique provides an assessment of actual gains or losses in productivity resulting from illness and disease. For many governments, interested as they are in maximizing productivity, that is an important feature of this method.

However, this method does have several disadvantages. Theoretically, willingness-to-pay is the correct measure, and the human capital approach may not even be a very good proxy for willingness to pay. Second, calculations based on human capital may undervalue those who are engaged in productive activities that do not earn a wage. The classic example of this is housewives. In early formulations of the human capital approach they were not given a value. In recognition of this fact, the theory has been revised to furnish estimates of how much they could make if engaged in other activities where wages are paid. (Alternatively, some researchers have estimated the market value of a housekeeper.) In other areas the theory remains rather simplistic. Elderly and retired people generally have little or no value attached to them, and much the same is true of unemployed people.

Willingness-to-pay is the standard concept of value in economics. Since morbidity and mortality include pain and suffering, this method provides a measure of intangible costs as well as indirect costs and direct costs paid by the patient. The willingness-to-pay approach is unique in its ability to provide estimates of intangible costs.

While willingness-to-pay is the theoretically correct measure, some commentators are concerned that it is a function of the ability to pay. Wealthier people obviously can pay more (and thus may be willing to pay more) for health than those with less money. In addition, willingness-to-pay may be more difficult to measure than the human capital approach. There are relatively few studies of peoples' willingness to pay for health care because researchers have, at least in the past, found it difficult to frame questions that people would answer about how much they would be willing to pay to avoid some degree of risk.[12,13] More research in this area is clearly indicated.

PERSPECTIVE

The last of the three dimensions of economic analysis of health care is point of view. The options embrace the viewpoints of society, the patient, and the payors for, or providers of, the services. The choice of perspective determines what things are regarded as costs, as well as their valuation. For instance, in the United Kingdom, hospitalization is charge-free for patients. Hence, from the patient's viewpoint, the only cost of hospitalization is his or her time or other intangibles. The hospital, however, has to pay for the patient's care; so, from the hospital's point of view, hospitalization of this patient does have a money cost.

Choice of perspective is not infrequently linked with issues of incentive, potential conflict of interest, and audience targeting. For instance, it may be shown that adding a particular drug to a hospital formulary will increase costs to the hospital pharmacy but reduce dispensing costs by requiring less time from skilled nursing staff. Hence, the hospital might realize an overall saving if this drug were adopted. On coming before the hospital formulary committee, however, the proposal might be rejected because pharmacy representatives assert that there are insufficient funds in the departmental budget to fund this (overall) cost-saving program.

This example highlights the problems of perspective, incentive, and targeting. The study takes a hospital-wide view of costs. The formulary committee, on the other hand, embodies various departmental perspectives. The pharmacy department, in particular, might not have the budget or the incentive to adopt the proposal. Since the evaluation concerned itself with overall cost to the hospital, it should rightly be referred to an individual or group who can take a similar broad view.

OTHER CONCEPTS

Sensitivity Analysis

Economic analyses of health care often must incorporate many assumptions about costs and benefits. These assumptions are duly entered on their respective sides of the balance sheet and a figure emerges that is described as the cost per QALY (or other measure of outcome). It is important to have some idea of the extent to which the result is affected by these assumptions. The process of testing the effect of changes in assumptions is called sensitivity analysis and involves recalculating the study results using alternative values for some of the variables to see if different sets of assumptions produce different conclusions.

Hence, sensitivity analysis has at least three functions. The first is to determine whether or not the preference for one program changes as the value of the variables used in the study change. Second, if this is the case, sensitivity analysis can identify the critical value of the variable where the preference of one program over another switches. Then, depending on which side of that critical value the variable is expected to fall, different choices or strategies may be recommended.

The third function of sensitivity analysis is to highlight those areas of the analysis where there is great uncertainty and where additional research may usefully be undertaken, such as identifying actual values for variables that have a critical effect on the outcome of an analysis.

Discount Rate

Assessments that look at costs and benefits over a long period of time must address the issue of discount rate. This concept embodies the fact that the costs and monetary benefits of a program may occur at different points in time, and that the value of money changes over time.

Costs incurred (and monetary benefits realized) now are generally greater than costs of similar nominal value incurred later -- if not used in the present the resources could be otherwise invested in the interim. Hence, it is necessary to express all costs and benefits at one point in time, usually the present. This is done by "bringing back" all the future costs (and monetary benefits) of a program and expressing them in terms of their present value (or in terms of future value if some time other than the present has been selected). A simple equation has been derived for this purpose:

$$\text{Present Value of Costs} = \sum_{T=0}^{N-1} \frac{C_T}{(1+R)^T}$$

Where:

C_T = costs at the time they are incurred

$(1 + R)^T$ = one plus the discount rate for costs (expressed as a decimal fraction of one), raised to the power of the time, T, during which costs are incurred

T = each of the N time periods (e.g., years) during which costs and benefits are incurred

Likewise: Present Value of Benefits $= \sum_{T=0}^{N-1} \dfrac{B_T}{(1 + R)^T}$

Where:

B_T = benefits at the time they are incurred

As an example of the discounting process, suppose that as part of a preventive health strategy $1,000 (inflation-adjusted) is spent per year for each of the next three years. Assume a discount rate of 5%. The present discounted value (PDV) equals the sum of $1,000 divided by 1.05 raised to the zero power (i.e., 1.0) plus $1,000 divided by 1.05 raised to the power of 1 (i.e., 1.05), plus $1,000 divided by 1.05 squared (i.e., 1.1025). This yields a total of $2,859.41. One way to think about this figure is as an annuity value: if this amount were invested today, it would be just possible to make the $1,000 payments in each of the next three years.

The discount rate is not just another term for inflation; even in an inflation-free world, some people will want to use money now (and be willing to pay for that privilege) while others will be willing to lend money now (and be paid for doing so). These different dispositions reflect time-preferences for money.

Two major issues emerge from any discussion of discounting. The first is what discount rate is appropriate.[14] Consideration of the discounting equation reveals that with a high discount rate, say 20%, monetary benefits accruing in the future are not worth much now. From the viewpoint of setting health care priorities, the effect of the discount rate can be significant. If, for instance, a preventive health program involving large present expenditure (i.e., high costs) yields benefits only in 20 years, and if the discount is 20%, then the present value of those benefits will be slight and may be seen as not justifying the costs. Treatment for acute problems that yield benefits immediately thus tend to be favored over preventive programs, in which the time to realization of benefits generally is longer. Lower discount rates imply that the value of money now is similar to that of money in the future. In such circumstances, projects that entail present expenditure in the hope of future benefits look more attractive.

The discount rate depends on people's preferences toward consumption now versus consumption in the future. Most developed countries employ a discount rate of about 5%, but due to the substantial impact discount rate can have on the outcome of an analysis, sensitivity analysis is usually undertaken using values around the chosen rate.

The second major issue in discounting is the debate over whether or not nonmonetary outcomes, such as gain in life expectancy, should be discounted at the same rate as monetary ones. While there is no clear-cut answer to this question, health economists in general agree that they should be discounted and that, at a minimum, if nondiscounted outcomes are reported, corresponding discounted outcomes should be reported as well.

Ethical Issues in Pharmacoeconomic Research

Ethical issues are raised when a value is placed on human life. However, these issues also arise in a number of other areas in cost-benefit and cost-effectiveness analysis. For example, while it has received little attention, they may arise when years of life are substituted for the value of life (in dollar terms) in cost-effectiveness analysis. If populations differ significantly in average life expectancy, interventions that might be justified in one population might not be justified in another. The ethical implications are greater when disparities in life expectancy are the result of discrimination.

Ethical issues also may be raised when two programs have similar costs and benefits, but distribute them differently across individuals in society. Suppose that the present value of the costs of two programs is $250,000 in each case, and that the present value of the benefits is a gain of 10 years of life. Suppose further that the difference between them is that in one the ten years accrue to one individual, while in the other these years are shared among five individuals. Analysis will indicate that the two programs are equivalent: the costs, effects, and the ratio of the cost-per-year-of-life-gained ($25,000) are all equal. However, if one form of distribution is considered fairer than the other (e.g., one that spreads benefits more evenly is fairer than one that provides greater benefits to a smaller number of individuals) or if one group is more deserving of that health care expenditure than another, there may be preferences for one program over another that will not be reflected in the economic analysis.

SUMMARY

In summary, economic assessments are multifaceted analyses that draw on a wide range of concepts. Among the key features are:

1. *Consistent application of explicitly stated rules*: Whatever the chosen type of analysis, this enables valid comparisons to be made with the assessments that use the same technique.
2. *Expressions of outcomes, such as the QALY, that enable the outcomes of different interventions to be compared.*
3. *Marginal costing*: In health care, it is very important to realize that the cost of additional services may well not be the same as the average cost of existing facilities.
4. *Discounting*: Estimates of discount rate and time to realization of benefits can have a big impact on the perceived financial viability of a project.

Ever increasing demand for health care has to be met from finite resources. It is this fact that underpins the growing need for systematic economic evaluations of health care. It is a mistake, however, to infer that "economics" means "budgetary cuts." The objective of health economic assessment is to get the best value for money, not to "save" money. Indeed, in the context of health care, the whole notion of "savings" may be a fallacy. Extending life is likely to result in increased calls on health care budgets as people live longer. Medical success is thus likely to lead to increases rather than decreases in health care budget and arguments about health care spending should be based on the value of these investments, rather than on purely financial grounds.

Decisions about allocation of resources are ultimately made at a political level. The function of economic evaluations is to ensure that these decisions are based on a rigorous assessment of the available options. As such, it is a means to an end, no more.

ACKNOWLEDGEMENT

This chapter was produced from a slide lecture kit developed under a grant from Merck Sharp & Dohme, International.

We gratefully acknowledge the comments and insights provided by John M. Eisenberg, M.D., M.B.A., but accept full responsibility for any errors.

REFERENCES

1. M. D. Nettelman, R. B. Jones, S. D. Roberts, P. Katz, E. Washington, R. S. Dittus, T. S. Quinn, Cost-effectiveness of culturing for Chlamydia trachomatis, *Ann. Intern. Med.* 105:189-96 (1986).

2.   C. Bombardier, J. Eisenberg, Looking into the crystal ball: Can we estimate the lifetime cost of rheumatoid arthritis?, *J. Rheumatol.* 12:201-204 (1984).

3.   A. Velez-Gil, D. Wilson, R. Nel Peleaz, A simplified system for surgical operation. The economics of treating hernia, *Surgery* 77:391-402 (1975).

4.   G. Torrance, Measurement of health state utilities for economic appraisal -- a review, *J Health Econ.* 5:1-30 (1986).

5.   J. Eisenberg, D. Kitz, Savings from outpatient antibiotic therapy for osteomyelitis, Economic analysis of a therapeutic strategy, *JAMA* 225:1584-8 (1986).

6.   J. M. Eisenberg, H. Koffer, S. A. Finkler, Economics analysis of a new drug: potential savings in hospital operating costs from the use of a once-daily regimen of a parenteral cephalosporin, *Rev. Infect. Dis.* 6:S909-23 (1984).

7.   W. F. McGhan, C. R. Rowland, J. L. Bootman, Cost-benefit and cost-effectiveness: methodologies for evaluating innovative pharmaceutical services, *Am. J. Hosp. Pharm.* 36:133-140 (1979).

8.   J. Paxinos, R. J. Hammel, W. L. Fritz, Contamination rates and costs associated with the use of four intermittent intravenous infusion systems, *Am. J. Hosp. Pharm.* 36:1497-503 (1978).

9.   S. Finkler, Cost finding for high-technology, high-cost services: current practices and a possible alternative, *Health Care Manage. Rev.* 5:17-29 (1980).

10.   S. V. Williams, S. A. Finkler, C. Murphy, J. M. Eisenberg, Improved cost allocation in case-mix accounting, *Med. Care* 20:450-9 (1982).

11.   T. W. Granneman, R. S. Brown, M. V. Pauly, Estimating hospital costs: a multiple output analysis, *J. Health Econ.* 5:107-27 (1986).

12.   M. S. Thompson, J. L. Read, M. Liang, Feasibility of willingness-to-pay measurement in chronic arthritis, *Med. Decis. Making* 4:195-215 (1984).

13.   M. Thompson, Willingness to pay and accept risks to cure chronic disease, *Am. J. Public Health* 76:392-96 (1986).

14.   R. C. Lind, A primer on the major issues relating to the discount rate for evaluating national energy options, *in*: "Discounting for time and risk in energy policy," R. C. Lind, et. al., eds., Resources for the Future, Inc., Washington, D.C. 21-94 (1982).

FURTHER READING

A. S. Detsky, and I. G. Naglie, A clinician's guide to cost-effectiveness analysis, *Ann Intern. Med.* 113:147-154 (1990).

M. F. Drummond, G. L. Stoddart, and G. W. Torrance, "Methods for the economic evaluation of health programmes," Oxford: Oxford University Press, (1987).

J. M. Eisenberg, H. Glick, and H. Koffer, Pharmacoeconomics: economic evaluation of pharmaceuticals, *in*: "Pharmacoepidemiology," B. L. Strom, ed., Churchill, Livingstone, N.Y., 325-350 (1989).

K. E. Warner, and B. R. Luce, "Cost-benefit and cost-effectiveness analysis in health care: principles, practice, and potential," Health Administration Press, Ann Arbor, MI, (1982).

N OF 1 RANDOMIZED TRIALS FOR INVESTIGATING NEW DRUGS

Gordon H. Guyatt, M.D.

Department of Medicine
and Department of Clinical Epidemiology and Biostatistics
McMaster University
Hamilton, Ontario, Canada

INTRODUCTION

Experimental studies of single subjects have been an important part of psychological research for some time.[1-3] The methodology is known as 'single case' or 'single subject' research, N = 1, or, as we shall call it, N of 1 trials. We have previously described how N of 1 randomized clinical trials (RCTs) may be used in medical practice to determine the optimum treatment of an individual patient and initiated an "N of 1 service" designed to assist clinicians who wish to conduct such a trial.[4] More recently, we have provided detailed guidelines for clinicians to conduct their own N of 1 RCTs.[5]

Whereas the previous work has been concerned with determining the most suitable treatment for single patients, the current paper explores the contributions N of 1 RCTs can make towards bridging the gap between early research findings in new drug development and the conduct of large sample clinical efficacy trials. We see the N of 1 approach being used in the early phases of the development of drugs designed to produce symptomatic benefit for chronic illness, which act quickly, and the biological action of which ends soon after withdrawal. While the approach could be modified to also consider frequently occurring side effects, our discussion will be almost entirely restricted to the assessment of anticipated therapeutic effects.

PROBLEMS IN DESIGNING LARGE-SAMPLE EFFICACY TRIALS

In large sample parallel group trials patients are assigned at random to one of the treatments under study, for example an investigational new drug treatment, a standard treatment, or placebo. The different treatment groups are followed for the response variable of interest. These trials are the standard approach to establishing drug efficacy, and to persuading regulatory agencies that a new medication should be placed on the market.

There are three major hurdles that need to be taken before such large sample parallel group trials of the efficacy and safety of a new drug can be undertaken. First, it must be determined whether the new drug shows sufficient promise to justify the initiation of a large clinical research program. Second, the patient population to be studied must be delineated. Third, the dose regimen to be used in the major trials must be established.

Decisions on these issues are generally based on findings from early clinical safety, tolerance, pharmacology and drug disposition studies in healthy volunteers and patients, augmented by ideas gained from initial small scale efficacy studies. These efficacy studies are often unmasked, and use baseline status or a historical reference group as a basis for comparison. Such studies tend to yield anecdotal information of questionable validity. Thus, when designing the first large-sample efficacy trial, investigators are faced with difficult decisions concerning both dose regimen and sample selection. They may gamble on a single dose, or take an approach that includes two or more different regimens for comparison. At the same time, they may hazard a guess at a suitable homogeneous target population of patients, or take a more conservative approach which includes a heterogeneous (possibly stratified) population.

If the investigators decide to gamble or guess and turn out to be substantially off the mark, the large-sample efficacy trial may provide misleading, or at least suboptimal, information. Nevertheless, the choice for gambling (on a single dose) and guessing (at the most likely population to benefit) is frequently made. The reason is that, even with a well-defined, homogeneous patient population, a parallel groups trial of a single dose of a new drug often requires large numbers of patients for adequate statistical power. Including a heterogeneous patient group in which drug effect on individual subgroups would have to be considered may make the sample size prohibitively larger. Similarly, the extra numbers required for inclusion of several different dosage regimens may well be considered unfeasible.

Even if, through good luck or sound judgement, the first large-sample efficacy trial demonstrates that the study population clearly benefits from the selected dosage of the new drug, important questions are likely to remain. Would as marked benefit have been obtained at lower doses, or would there be additional benefit with higher doses? Are there subgroups of patients who are particularly responsive or resistant to the new drug? Because of the difficulty of determining the profiles of responsive and drug resistant subpopulations of patients, even several successive rounds of large-sample parallel groups trials may fail to provide clear cut answers to these questions.

THE ROLE OF N OF 1 RCTS

N of 1 trials share many features in common with traditional cross-over trials. The fundamental difference between the N of 1 approach and traditional cross-over trials is their primary purpose: N of 1 trials attempt to establish effects in an individual, cross-over trials attempt to establish effects in a group. As a secondary goal, one may use a cross-over trial to examine individual responses. By the same token, one may analyze a series of N of 1 trials with a similar design as a multiple cross-over trial (i.e., a large sample trial in which each patient is repeatedly exposed to experimental and control conditions). However, the N of 1 trial will be designed so that individual effects can be reliably detected; the cross-over trial will be designed so that individual estimates of response are imprecisely estimated but the magnitude of the average group effect can be efficiently determined. Variability of individual response precludes strong inference regarding benefit in an individual from a single exposure to experimental and control conditions. To confidently classify an individual as a responder or a non-responder multiple exposures are required.

In some therapeutic indications, the problems faced by investigators may be over-come by including a series of N of 1 RCTs. These trials will permit the identification of responders and non-responders, and an estimate of the proportion of patients in each category. They may also make it possible to determine the optimal dosage regimen for individual patients. The availability of this type of information makes the design of large-scale parallel groups trials less problematic.

These benefits can be obtained if the condition under study is chronic, relatively stable, and the new treatment begins to act within days (or at most, a couple of weeks) and ceases acting after discontinuation over a similar time frame. These include conditions such as chronic airflow limitation, stable angina, chronic pain syndromes (including chronic arthritis), irritable bowel syndrome, movement disorders such as Parkinson's disease, and many others. N of 1 RCTs are unlikely to be useful when major outcomes that occur over the long-term (including death, or major morbidity such as stroke) are the end-points of interest.

THE ROLE OF N OF 1 RCTS: A SPECIFIC EXAMPLE

To illustrate the role of N of 1 RCTs in drug development, we will describe a series of N of 1 studies we have conducted in patients with fibrositis. Fibrositis is a syndrome characterized by generalized aches and pains, morning stiffness, fourteen body sites at which patients are particularly sensitive to pressure (tender points), and an associated sleep disturbance.[6] While one conventional randomized trial has shown that on average patients with fibrositis improve with amitriptyline[7], for the exposition which follows we ask the reader to view amitriptyline as a promising, but not yet formally proven, treatment for fibrositis.

Under these circumstances questions of interest would include the following: does the drug really work in anyone? what is the optimal dose? how quickly does the drug work? what proportion of fibrositis patients respond? can patient characteristics that are predictive of response or non-response be identified?

Unmasked therapeutic trials may introduce varying amounts of bias depending on the possibility of cointervention, and the extent to which subjective factors can influence measurement of outcome. For instance, in a trial of a surgical therapy for a medically untreatable condition in which mortality is the primary outcome, little bias is likely to be introduced by the absence of masking. However, in the context in which N of 1 trials are likely to be useful (i.e., when the goal of therapy is to ameliorate symptoms) patient and physician expectations and the placebo effect are very likely to influence measurement of treatment targets.[4,5] Biases introduced by these factors are generally likely to favor a conclusion that the new treatment is beneficial. Thus, a false positive conclusion (concluding the drug works when it doesn't) is far more likely than a false negative conclusion (concluding the drug does not work when in fact it does). Accordingly, it might be reasonable to conduct formal N of 1 studies only on patients with apparent responses in unmasked trials.

The decision concerning the initial dose to be tested is to some extent arbitrary; one approach would be to begin with the smallest dose that could produce a therapeutic effect. Another important decision is the period duration. One wishes to allow enough time for a full therapeutic response to occur and to be adequately assessed (and for the response to wear off). On the other hand, the shorter the periods, the more efficient the trial is generally likely to be. When investigating a new drug one is likely to begin with only a very general estimate of the likely onset (and termination) of treatment effect. One strategy for dealing with this dilemma is to begin using the longest treatment periods that are feasible (for most N of 1 trials, this will be somewhere between four and six weeks per period). If one finds evidence of a rapid onset and termination of action the period duration can be shortened for subsequent trials.

We employed these strategies in our N of 1 trials of amitriptyline in fibrositis. Patients with clinical findings suggestive of fibrositis were prescribed 10 mg. of amitriptyline to be taken each day at bed time in an unmasked trial. In patients who did not respond the dose was increased gradually up to 50 mg. per day. Those who reported improvement on the initial or subsequent dose were enrolled in an N of 1 RCT at the dose that gave an apparent benefit in the unmasked trial. In the N of 1 RCTs, patients received pairs of treatment periods (each pair included one period each of active drug and placebo, in random order); patient and clinician were kept masked to allocation, and treatment targets were monitored.

We began with treatment periods of four weeks duration. Every patient was asked to rate the severity of seven symptoms (including aches and pains, quality of sleep, and headaches), each on a seven point scale, at weekly intervals. The results of one of the first trials, a study using 10 mg. of amitriptyline in a 47 year old woman with symptoms of five years duration, are depicted in Figure 1. Each data point represents the mean severity score for the seven symptoms which the patient rated each week. Our experience with the seven point scales suggests that the minimal clinically important difference is approximately half a point per question. That is, if patients' scores increase (higher scores representing better function) by at least a mean of half a point per question, patients report a noticeable improvement in function which is important in their daily lives. Bearing this in mind, the results of the trial suggest a small but clinically

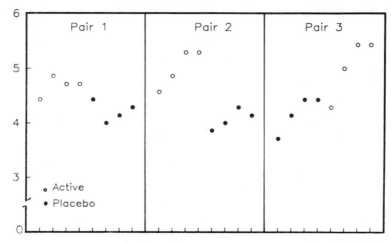

Figure 1.   Results of an N of 1 RCT in a patient with fibrositis. Horizontal axis is
time, vertical axis is mean symptom score.

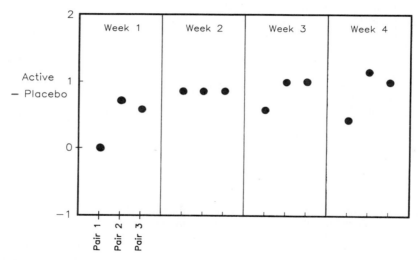

Figure 2.   Results of an N of RCT in a patient with fibrositis: data presented
separately for weeks 1, 2, and 3 of each period.   Vertical axis is mean
symptom score on active drug minus mean symptom score on placebo.

important treatment effect of amitriptyline. They also suggest that the treatment acts
quickly after it is instituted, and ceases to act shortly after being discontinued. Another
way of examining the rapidity of onset of action is depicted in Figure 2. Here, the mean
treatment effect is calculated separately for each week, i.e., for each pair of treatment
periods. In other words, the first week on placebo is compared to the first week on active
drug, the second week on placebo to the second week on active drug, and so on. If, for
example, the drug had an effect that took two weeks to appear, one would expect to see a
mean effect of 0 for the first two weeks, the effect appearing for only the latter two weeks
of the treatment periods. The fact that the treatment effect is consistent across all four
weeks supports a rapid onset (and termination) of drug action.
        One can apply a statistical analysis to these results. Using a "sign test" based on
the binomial distribution and assuming there is no treatment difference, the probability of
three consecutive pairs of treatment periods favoring active treatment is 1/8 or 0.125

(one-sided test). If one is willing to accept the assumptions required (discussed in the section concerning study design and statistical analysis which follows), one can analyze the data using the paired t-test. The mean difference between active and placebo periods is 0.78; a paired t test of the differences between matched active and placebo periods shows a t value of 4.90. With two degrees of freedom, the associated two-sided p value is 0.039. One can use the same approach to generate confidence intervals. In this case, the 90% confidence intervals suggest that the treatment effect is likely to vary between 0.3 and 1.2 points in this patient.

The results of an N of 1 RCT in a second patient, a 54 year old woman with symptoms of two years duration, are depicted in Figure 3. Here one sees a slightly larger, consistent, treatment effect. The statistical analysis showed a t value of 4.78 with two degrees of freedom, an associated p value of 0.041, and a 90% confidence interval of 0.53 to 2.20. The results again suggest a rapid onset and offset of drug action (Figure 3). This conclusion is further supported by an examination of the individual treatment effects associated with the four weeks of the study (Figure 4). Having established that amitriptyline can have a rapid onset of action in fibrositis patients, we used two week treatment periods in our subsequent N of 1 RCTs in this investigation.

Approximately one third of new referrals with fibrositis have shown apparent benefit from an unmasked trial of amitriptyline. Consequently, in two thirds of the patients the medication was discontinued without an N of 1 RCT being conducted. To date, we have conducted 14 N of 1 RCTs in fibrositis patients in whom an unmasked trial suggested a benefit from amitriptyline. Of these, 6 have confirmed the treatment effect (showing consistently better function on active than placebo, with a paired t-test on the data yielding a value of < 0.05). Four have refuted the results of the unmasked trial (clinically important difference in favour of active treatment found in none of three pairs of treatment periods). In another four patients, variability in response was sufficient to preclude a definitive conclusion; however, the results of three of these trials suggested that amitriptyline was of no benefit, while the fourth showed a trend suggesting effectiveness (p = 0.10). The doses used in the six positive trials included 10 mg., 20 mg., 25 mg., and 50 mg. per day. It is thus evident that amitriptyline can be effective in doses that might have been considered homeopathic. It is not necessary to give all patients the standard dose of 50 mg. per day which was used in the positive parallel groups RCT[7]; smaller doses may avoid anticholinergic side effects associated with amitriptyline.

N OF 1 RCTS FOR NEW DRUG DEVELOPMENT: THE GENERAL CASE

In relating the foregoing examples to the general use of N of 1 RCTs in drug development we will deal in turn with the following seven issues: the role of unmasked trials of medication, determining the rapidity of onset of drug action, optimizing dose, measuring outcome, study design and statistical analysis, assessing potential drug impact, and predicting response (Table 1).

The Role of Unmasked Trials of Medication

The studies we have described were not done as part of an investigation of amitriptyline in fibrositis, but rather to sort out whether therapy was warranted in individual patients. If one were conducting a systematic investigation of a new drug, the assumption that an unmasked trial showing no apparent benefit excludes a clinically important treatment effect could be tested by conducting formal N of 1 studies in patients who initially fail to improve. If a number of such trials confirm the assumption, formal N of 1 RCTs could be restricted to patients showing apparent benefit in unmasked trials. Restricting formal N of 1 RCTs to those who had shown an apparent response in an unmasked trial would improve the efficiency of the investigation.

Determining the Rapidity of Onset and Termination of Action

We concluded that the onset and termination of treatment effect was rapid after two N of 1 RCTs in which an advantage of drug over placebo was evident during the first week of each four week treatment period. Although subsequent studies using two week

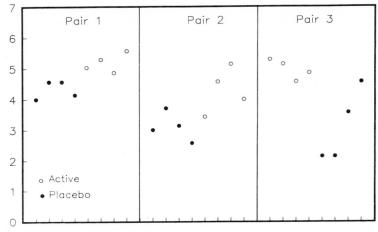

Figure 3.   Results of an N of 1 RCT in a patient with fibrositis. Horizontal axis is time, vertical axis is mean symptom score.

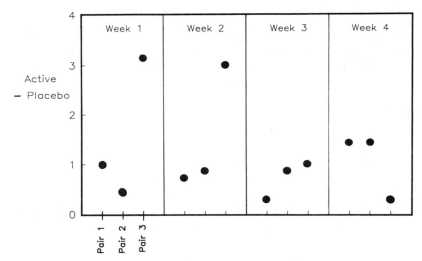

Figure 4.   Results of an N of RCT in a patient with fibrositis: data presented separately for weeks 1, 2, and 3 of each period. Vertical axis is mean symptom score.

periods have confirmed this impression, investigators studying a previously untested drug may wish to have further evidence before shortening treatment periods.

Optimizing Dose

In our fibrositis studies, we were willing to allow unmasked dose titration aiming at a response in the individual patient. Unmasked trials are open to the play of a number of biases which could lead to inaccurate assessment of optimal doses. One of many alternative approaches would be to begin an N of 1 trial with the lowest dose which may produce a treatment effect. If the first pair of treatment periods (in which active and placebo would be compared, the order determined by random allocation) showed no clear

Table 1.   Issues and Opportunities Using N of 1 Trials in Drug Development

1)   The role of unmasked trials of medication

Does a negative unmasked trial exclude benefit?

2)   Determining the rapidity of onset of drug action

How quickly does the drug begin to act, and cease acting?

3)   Optimising dose

What is the "best" dose? Does it differ between patients?

4)   Measurement of Outcome

What outcomes are most influenced by the new drug?

5)   Study Design and Statistical analysis

What designs and analytic tools are available for planning N of 1 RCTs, and for evaluating their results?

6)   Interpreting the Results of N of 1 RCTs.

What a priori criteria should be established for classifying a trial as definitively positive, definitively negative, or indefinite?

7)   Assessing potential drug impact

Will the drug have a significant impact on the disease?

8)   Predicting response

Are there features that discriminate between responders and non-responders?

cut difference a higher dose could be used in the next pair of treatment periods. The process could continue until side effects were noted, the highest acceptable dose was reached, or a clear cut difference between active and placebo observed.   Treatment effects could be confirmed by conducting additional pairs of treatment periods on the apparently favorable dose. This approach would not only help determine the optimal dose, but would reveal whether this optimal dose differed in different patients, an issue that would be very difficult to elucidate by parallel group studies. In addition, it would be possible to modify the doses used after only a few trials, if a high incidence of toxicity (use lower doses), or a low incidence of response (use higher doses) were found. One alternative design would include a series of masked periods on differing doses, one of which would be a placebo. Finally, one could conduct (for instance) five N of 1 RCTs on each of three doses and, depending on the results, modify the doses used for subsequent N of 1 RCTs.

A final point is the issue of harmful drug effects, for which the investigator must look carefully. If a drug is of benefit in half of the intended population, but has major deleterious effects in the other half, it is unlikely that the manufacturer will wish to proceed with drug development, unless reliable predictors of response were found.

Measurement of Outcome

In the initial study of a new drug, investigators may be uncertain about the outcomes on which to focus. This is particularly true if the primary outcomes relate to patients' symptoms, and if the condition being treated results in a spectrum of problems. For example, a drug for fibrositis may have differential impact on the aches and pains, the sleep disturbance, or the associated symptoms of headache and bowel disturbance. These differences may become apparent in initial positive N of 1 RCTs, giving the investigator an opportunity to shift the focus of outcome measurement to the areas most likely to benefit.

We have observed an example of this using N of 1 RCTs to study a new drug in patients with senile dementia. While our initial outcomes focused almost exclusively on cognitive dysfunction and associated deficits in performance, we found after only two N of 1 RCTs that patients reported changes in aspects of behavior (alertness, responsiveness, willingness to cooperate) during the studies. We were thus able to modify our outcomes to measure aspects of behavior more thoroughly in subsequent trials. This experience highlights the flexibility that can be introduced through using N of 1 RCTs in the initial investigation of new drugs.

Study Design and Statistical Analysis

While we have dealt in detail with a study design that uses matched pairs of treatment periods, other classical experimental designs such as randomized blocks and latin squares can be readily adapted to N of 1 RCTs. For each of these designs, a number of options for statistical analysis are available. These include non-parametric or distribution free methods, (such as the sign test based on the binomial distribution), and parametric methods collectively known as 'analysis of variance' of which the t-test is a special case.

In the fibrositis example, we saw that the smallest one-sided p-value that can occur with the application of the binomial distribution to the data from the design with three matched pairs equals 0.125. In contrast, the paired t-test permits much smaller values (in fact, all values between 0 and 1 are possible). A second benefit of the paired t-test is that is often more powerful; that is, if a treatment difference does exist, the paired t-test is often more likely to achieve statistical significance than the sign test based on the binomial distribution.

The price that must be paid for these advantages is that, whereas the randomization alone is sufficient to guarantee the validity of the sign test, other requirements have to be met for the paired t-test to be strictly valid. The differences between the observations within each pair of treatment periods must be normally distributed with consistent mean and variance from pair to pair; further, these differences must be independent. In the chronic conditions for which the N of 1 approach is most appropriate serial dependency, which occurs when values tend to drift upward and downward during good and bad phases, is likely to be present. However, with randomized designs such as the randomized blocks and latin square designs, approximate validity is assured if the treatment effects remain constant over time.[8] Another way to express this requirement is to say that the value of the response variable in each of the treatment periods equals the value that would have been observed if one and the same treatment had been given throughout the study (say treatment A) plus a fixed value constant over all periods due to the actual treatment given in the period (say treatment B). This fixed value represents the systematic difference of interest between treatments A and B. With continuous response variables, this additivity requirement may well hold true to a good first approximation.

Fortunately, serial dependency is not as big a problem as it is sometimes made out to be. In an examination of the data from approximately 500 N of 1 data sets which have appeared in the psychological literature, Huitema[9] found no evidence of autocorrelation which would call the validity of analysis of variance methods into question. Furthermore, our own analysis of 17 N of 1 RCTs showed no evidence of clinically or statistically significant autocorrelation.[10]

In those cases where non-parametric methods of data analysis are indicated, the number of different treatment assignments that are possible and with it the number of different achievable p-values can be increased enormously by randomly varying the lengths of the successive treatment periods. A good account of the possibilities is given by Edgington.[11] Alternatively, randomization of treatments to periods can be unconstrained, or constrained only so far as to avoid extreme distributions.[11]

This summary of the design and analytical possibilities for the conduct of N of 1 RCTs is, by necessity, brief and superficial. More detailed discussion by other authors[1-3,8] and our own more detailed overview[10], can be found elsewhere.

Interpreting the Results of N of 1 RCTs

An investigator who has conducted a series of N of 1 RCTs may elect to simply describe the results, and conclude whether the treatment is working based on a graphical display of the data. However, the investigator must be aware of the potential for bias in interpreting N of 1 RCT results. There are three possible outcomes of an N of 1 RCT comparing a drug to placebo: the drug is clearly of benefit, clearly not of benefit (including the possibility of a harmful effect), or the results do not permit a definitive conclusion. Subjectivity in assessing findings can be decreased if criteria for each of these outcomes is specified before the series of N of 1 RCTs is begun. Statistical analysis can be useful in this regard. For example, one has the opportunity to use the conventional criterion for a definitive positive trial ($p \leq 0.05$) or other criteria which seem more appropriate (for example, based on confidence intervals).

Even if one has set a priori criteria, a misleading picture can emerge if these criteria are not set appropriately. Too lenient criteria will result in excessive type 1 error; too strict criteria will lead to large type 2 error. As described below in our discussion of assessing potential drug impact, a pharmaceutical company may set criteria according to factors such as the potential size of the market, the number of competitors, and the production costs of the new agent.

Assessing Potential Drug Impact

When a number of N of 1 trials have been conducted, one is in a position to evaluate the potential impact of the new medication. We found that approximately one quarter of the patients with a clinical diagnosis of fibrositis showed true benefit from amitriptyline. In a condition as common as fibrositis, when the drug (at the doses used) is inexpensive and non-toxic, a 25% response rate suggests an important role for the medication. If only one out of 20 patients has a positive N of 1 RCT, a drug is probably not worth developing further; if 15 out of 20 respond, one clearly has an important new treatment. Between such extremes, the decision concerning further study will depend on factors such as the prevalence of the condition being treated, its associated morbidity, the expense and toxicity of the treatment, the availability of other effective treatments, and the likelihood of correctly predicting response. We should note that in a condition which results in severe morbidity and for which there is no other treatment, an inexpensive and non-toxic drug might be worth developing and using even if only a small proportion of patients gained a clinically important benefit.

If N of 1 RCTs suggest further study is warranted, the results can help in planning subsequent investigations. For example, sample size for a parallel groups study can be more accurately decided by information from prior N of 1 RCTs concerning both within-person variability over time and between patient heterogeneity of treatment response. The lower the response rate in preceding N of 1 RCTs, the larger the sample size required in subsequent parallel group designs.

Predicting Response

N of 1 RCTs can also help determine eligibility criteria for subsequent studies. The precise identification of responders and non-responders allows powerful examination of predictors of response. If there is very little overlap between responders and non-responders (for example, if virtually all people over 50 respond, and all those under 50 do not) a small number of N of 1 RCTs will allow identification of variables associated with response. If a larger number of N of 1 RCTs have been completed, weaker predictors may also be identified. If the number of trials is large enough, one may consider the use of statistical methods, for example logistic regression models, to determine the independent contribution of a set of variables in differentiating responders from non-responders.

Identifying variables associated with response is important for clinicians in deciding when to use a drug. In addition, the ability of N of 1 RCTs to precisely define responders may provide a solution to one of the major dilemmas facing those investigating a new drug: choosing the population for the first large-sample parallel groups RCT.

CONCLUSIONS

N of 1 RCTs have an important role to play in the development of new drugs. Information regarding rapidity of onset and termination of drug action, the optimal dose, the outcomes on which to focus, and predictors of response may be obtained most efficiently using N of 1 RCTs. The ultimate impact of a new medication can be assessed early on in the process of clinical testing.

The major limitation of N of 1 RCTs is that they are most appropriate if the condition under study is chronic and relatively stable, for drugs which manifest an effect on a clinically important treatment target within days to several weeks and whose effect is reversed over a similar time period when withdrawn. The arguments presented here are theoretical; N of 1 RCTs have not as yet played a major role in the development of any drug. As a result, the best ways of conducting N of 1 RCTs in this setting remain to be established. Questions include the necessity for double-masked N of 1 RCTs when a preliminary unmasked trial in the same patient is negative, the optimal number of pairs of treatment periods, the choice of design, the relative merits of fixed versus variable period length and parametric versus non-parametric analysis. However, the method has sufficient promise that these questions should be addressed through use of N of 1 RCTs as an important part of the strategy for testing of new drugs.

REFERENCES

1. T. R. Kratchwill, ed, "Single subject research: strategies forevaluating change," Academic Press, Orlando, Fla (1978).
2. D. H. Barlow, Hersen M., "Single case experimental designs: strategies for studying behavior change," Pergamon Press 2nd ed, New York (1984).
3. A. E. Kazdin, "Single-case research designs: methods for clinical and applied settings," Oxford University Press, New York (1982).
4. G. H. Guyatt, D. Sackett, D. W. Taylor, J. Chong, R. Roberts, and S. Pugsley, Determining Optimal Therapy - Randomized Trials in Individual Patients, *N Engl J Med.* 314:889-892 (1986).
5. G. H. Guyatt, D. L. Sackett, J. D. Adachi, and et. al., A Clinician's guide for conducting randomized trials in individual patients, *Can Med Ass J.* 139:497-503 (1988).
6. S. Clark, S. M. Campbell, M. E. Forehand, and et. al., Clinical characteristics of fibrositis, *Arthritis Rheum.* 28:132-137 (1985).
7. S. Carette, G. A. McCain, D. A. Bell, and A. G. Fam, Evaluation of amitriptyline in primary fibrositis, *Arthritis Rheum.* 29:655-659 (1986).
8. O. Kempthorne, "The design and analysis of experiments," John Wiley and Sons Incorporated, London, (1967).
9. B. E. Huitema, Autocorrelation in applied behavior analysis: a myth, *Behav Assessment.* 7:107-118 (1985).
10. R. S. Roberts, R. Jaeschke, J. Keller, and G. H. Guyatt, Design and analysis of N of 1 randomized trials: the options, Submitted for publication.
11. E. S. Edgington, Statistics and single case analysis, *Prog Behav Modif.* 16:83-119 (1984).

MEASURING HEALTH-RELATED QUALITY OF LIFE IN CLINICAL TRIALS

Gordon H. Guyatt, M.D.

Department of Medicine
and Department of Clinical Epidemiology
   and Biostatistics
McMaster University
Hamilton, Ontario, Canada

During the last decade, the importance of measuring aspects of health status related to patients' function and subjective experience has become increasingly recognized. The methods available for measuring how patients feel, and how they function, have become more sophisticated. The term "quality of life" has appeared as a label for the measurement of physical and emotional (as opposed to biochemical and physiological) function.[1] Of course, quality of life is influenced by many factors other than one's health (such as one's income, job satisfaction, social opportunities); what health researchers are interested in is "health-related quality of life" (HRQL). We will use HRQL to refer to the wide variety of subjective experiences (including symptoms, physical function, and emotional function) which are related to health.

One may be interested in the impact of a disease or condition on HRQL[2,3], the profile of dysfunction in a particular population[4], or the relation between HRQL and prognosis.[5] For clinicians, and for the pharmaceutical industry, one crucial arena for HRQL measurement is determining the impact of medical interventions on how patients feel, and how they function. Readers of clinical journals are starting to face clinical trials in which HRQL is the primary outcome.[6-8] The purpose of the present paper is to suggest a taxonomy for HRQL measures, and to review the possible approaches to measurement of HRQL in clinical trials and their relative merits. The present discussion, which is built on the contributions of previous authors in this area [for instance,[1,9-14]], focuses on the empirical performance of HRQL measures in clinical trials, rather than the theoretical framework upon which the measures are based. A summary of the strengths and weaknesses of the HRQL measures is presented in Table 1.

NECESSARY ATTRIBUTES OF A QUALITY-OF-LIFE MEASUREMENT INSTRUMENT

Before proceeding to a more detailed discussion of the approaches to HRQL measurement in pharmaceutical trials it is necessary to briefly review the attributes inherent in any useful instrument. There are two essential attributes: validity and responsiveness.

Validity

Validity or accuracy is a necessary property of any useful test or instrument: the instrument must be measuring what it is supposed to measure.[15-17]

Table 1.   Taxonomy of Measures of Health-Related Quality of Life in
                Pharmaceutical Trials

Approach	Strengths	Weaknesses
Generic Instruments		
Health Profile	-Single instrument -Established reliability and validity -Detects differential effects on different aspects of health status -Comparison across interventions, conditions possible	-May not focus adequately on area of interest -May not be responsive
Utility Measurement	-Single number representing net impact on HRQL -Cost-utility analysis possible	-Difficulty determining utility values -Doesn't allow examination of effect on different aspects of HRQL -May not be responsive
Specific Instruments	-Clinically sensible -May be more responsive	-Doesn't allow cross condition comparisons -May be limited in terms of populations and interventions
Disease specific		
Population specific		
Function specific		
Condition or Problem specific		

Establishing accuracy is relatively easy if there is a criterion or gold standard to which the new instrument can be compared. However, there is no gold standard measure for HRQL. As a result, the validity of HRQL measures is established by specifying the domain or dimension one wishes to measure, and the expected relations between that domain or dimension and other variables. Thus, one assembles empirical evidence to support the inference that a particular instrument is measuring what it is supposed to measure. Many questionnaires used in clinical trials rely on face validity: intuitively, the questions appear to relate to aspects of HRQL. Unfortunately, it is difficult to be certain of what the results of such ad hoc instruments mean. For example, questionnaires asking patients if their function improved after a rehabilitation program may be measuring satisfaction with the program, rather than HRQL. The validity of a questionnaire must be established before it can be applied as a meaningful outcome measure in pharmaceutical trials.

Responsiveness

Investigators want to detect any clinically important changes in HRQL, even if those changes are small. Responsiveness (or sensitivity to change) refers to the instrument's ability to detect clinically important change. An instrument's responsiveness is determined by two properties.[18] First, to be responsive it should be reproducible; that is, repetition in stable subjects should yield more or less the same result. Second, it must register changes in score when subjects' HRQL improves or deteriorates; this property can be called changeability. If an instrument's responsiveness is unproved, and a controlled trial in which the instrument is used is negative, there remain two interpretations. First, the treatment doesn't work; second, the instrument is not responsive. Thus, when beginning a trial, it is desirable to use a questionnaire which has proved responsive in previous related investigations.

All HRQL measures, irrespective of the approach used, must be reproducible, valid, and responsive to be useful as outcome measures in pharmaceutical trials.

TAXONOMY OF MEASURES OF QUALITY OF LIFE

Generic Instruments

Generic instruments are applicable to a wide variety of populations. Their broad applicability is, in general, derived from their coverage of the complete spectrum of function, disability, and distress that is relevant to HRQL. Generic instruments can be divided into two major classes: Health Profiles and Utility Measures.

Health Profiles

Health profiles are single instruments which measure different aspects of HRQL. Health profiles share a common scoring system, and can be aggregated into a small number of scores and sometimes into a single score (in which case, it may be referred to as an index). As generic measures, they are designed for use in a wide variety of conditions. For example, one of the most popular health profiles, the Sickness Impact Profile (SIP)[19], contains 12 "categories" which can be aggregated into two dimensions and five independent categories, and also into a single overall score. The SIP has been used in studies of cardiac rehabilitation[20], total hip joint arthroplasty[21], and treatment of back pain.[8] In addition to the Sickness Impact Profile, there are a number of other health profiles available: the Nottingham Health Profile[22], the McMaster Health Index Questionnaire[23], and a collection of related instruments developed by the Rand Corporation for their health insurance study.[24]

Although each health profile attempts to measure all important aspects of HRQL, they may divide HRQL in different categories or dimensions. For example, the McMaster Health Index Questionnaire follows the World Health Organization approach and identifies three dimensions: Physical, Emotional, and Social. The Sickness Impact Profile includes a Physical dimension (with categories of ambulation, mobility, and body care and movement), a Psychosocial dimension (with categories including social interaction and emotional behaviour), and five independent categories including eating, work, home management, sleep and rest, and recreations and pastimes.

Health profiles offer a number of advantages to the clinical investigator. Their reproducibility and validity have been established, often in a variety of populations. They allow determination of the effects of the intervention on different aspects of HRQL without necessitating the use of multiple instruments (and thus saving both the investigator's and the patient's time). Because they are designed for a wide variety of conditions, one can potentially compare the effects on HRQL of different interventions in different diseases. They can be used in a cost-effectiveness analysis, in which the cost of an intervention in dollars is related to its outcome in natural units. For example, one could examine the incremental cost necessary to produce a five point improvement in score on the Sickness Impact Profile.

Health Profiles also have limitations. They may not focus adequately on the aspects of HRQL of specific interest to the investigator. For example, we recently encountered an investigator interested in measuring the effects of antiarrhythmic therapy on HRQL. None of the 136 items in the Sickness Impact Profile relate directly to symptoms which may be ameliorated by anti-arrhythmic therapy: palpitations, pre-syncope, and syncope. Inadequate focus on the HRQL issues of a specific trial is likely to result in an unresponsive instrument which may miss small but still clinically important changes in HRQL.[25,26] On the other hand, when the intervention is likely to have an impact on aspects of HRQL included in a health profile, responsiveness may be adequate. For example, at least some of the Sickness Impact Profile dimensions have detected differences between intervention and control groups in randomized trials of cardiac rehabilitation[20], and amputation versus limb sparing surgery in soft tissue sarcoma.[27] Health profiles may detect unexpected, but important, effects.

A final limitation of health profiles is that if they do not yield a single score, their usefulness in cost-effectiveness analysis is limited. If they do yield a single score, but that score is not preferentially weighted, they cannot be used in costutility analysis. This issue is discussed further in the following section.

Utility Measurement

Utility measures of HRQL are derived from economic and decision theory, and reflect the preferences of patients for treatment process and outcome. HRQL is measured holistically as a single number along a continuum from death (0.0) to full health (1.0). Use of utility measures in clinical trials requires serial measurement of the utility of the patient's HRQL throughout the study.

There are two fundamental approaches to utility measurement in clinical trials. One is to ask patients a number of questions about their function. On the basis of their responses patients are classified into one of a number of categories. Each category has a utility value associated with it, the utility having been established in previous ratings by another group (such as a random sample of the general population). This approach characterizes a widely used instrument called the Quality of Well-Being Scale.[10,11,15]

The second approach is to ask patients to make a single rating which takes into account all aspects of their HRQL.[12] There are many ways this rating can be made. The standard gamble asks subjects to choose between their own health state and a gamble in which they may die immediately or achieve full health for the remainder of their lives. Using the standard gamble, patients' utility or HRQL is determined by the choices they make as the probabilities of immediate death or full health are varied. The standard gamble has the advantage of fulfilling the fundamental axioms of utility theory as developed by von Neumann and Morgenstern.[12] A simplified and more widely used technique is the time trade off in which subjects are asked about the number of years in their present health state they would be willing to trade off for a shorter life span in full health.[12]

A major advantage of utility measurement is its amenability to cost-utility analysis. In cost-utility analysis the cost of an intervention is related to the number of quality-adjusted life-years (QUALYs) gained through application of the intervention. For example, it has been estimated (though not on the basis of data from clinical trials in which utilities were measured) that the cost per QUALY gained is $4,500 for neonatal intensive care for 1,000 to 1,499 gram neonates[12] and $54,000 for hospital hemodialysis (both figures in 1983 dollars).[12] Such comparisons provide a basis for allocation of scarce resources among health-care programs. Results from the utility approach may thus be of particular interest to program evaluators and health-policy decision makers.

Utility measurement also has limitations. Utilities can vary depending on how they are obtained, raising questions of the validity of any single measurement.[28,29] Differences between scores obtained from standard gamble versus time trade-off methods are, however, seldom very dramatic. Utilities do not allow the investigator to determine what aspects of HRQL are responsible for changes in utility. On the other hand, subjects provide a holistic rating taking both treatment and side effects into account. Finally, utilities at least potentially share the disadvantage of health profiles in that they may not be responsive to small, but still clinically important, changes.

However, utility measurement has proved responsive in at least one pharmaceutical trial. In a double-blind randomized trial of auranofin versus placebo in rheumatoid arthritis both the Quality of Well-Being scale and a measure based on the time trade-off proved highly responsive (indeed, more so than traditional measures such as the number of tender or swollen joints).[30] This trial allowed direct comparison between various measures of HRQL, and thus provides a model for the sort of study which will allow determination of the optimal methods for measuring HRQL in clinical trials.

Specific Instruments

An alternative approach to HRQL measurement is to focus on aspects of health status which are specific to the area of primary interest.[17] The rationale for this approach lies in its potential for increased responsiveness which may result from including only important aspects of HRQL which are relevant to the patients being studied. The instrument may even focus on problems which are specific to the individual patient.[31]

The instrument may be specific to the disease (instruments for chronic lung disease, or for rheumatoid arthritis); specific to a population of patients (instruments designed to measure the HRQL of the frail elderly, who are afflicted with a wide variety of different diseases); specific to a certain function (questionnaires which examine emotional or sexual function); or they may be specific to a given condition or problem (such as pain) which may be caused by a variety of underlying pathologies. Within a single condition, the questionnaire may differ depending on the intervention. For example, while success of a disease modifying agent in rheumatoid arthritis should result in improved HRQL by enabling a patient to increase performance of physically stressful activities of daily living, occupational therapy may achieve improved HRQL by encouraging family members to take over activities formerly accomplished with difficulty by the patient. Appropriate disease-specific HRQL outcome measures should reflect this difference.

In addition to the likelihood of improved responsiveness, specific measures have the advantage of relating closely to areas routinely explored by the physician. For example, a disease-specific measure of HRQL in chronic lung disease focuses on dyspnea on day to day activities, fatigue, and areas of emotional dysfunction including frustration and impatience.[31] Specific measures may therefore appear clinically sensible to the physician.

Disease-specific measures have been developed for many conditions, including cardiovascular disease[32], chronic lung disease[31,33], arthritis[34,35], and cancer.[36-37] Specific instruments can be constructed to reflect the "single state" (how tired have you been: very tired, somewhat tired, full of energy) or a "transition" (how has your tiredness been: better, the same, worse).[38] Morbidity, including events such as recurrent myocardial infarction, can be integrated into a specific measures.[32] Guidelines for constructing specific measures are available.[17,38] Disease-specific instruments have proved useful in clinical trials.[6,31,32]

The disadvantages of specific measures is that they are (deliberately) not comprehensive, and cannot be used to compare across conditions or, at times, even across programmes. Determining whether specific measures increase responsiveness and clinical credibility sufficient to warrant their use will require head-to-head comparisons of different approaches in the setting of randomized controlled trials.[30]

USE OF MULTIPLE QUALITY-OF-LIFE MEASURES IN CLINICAL TRIALS

Clinical investigators are not restricted to using a single instrument in their trials. Much remains to be learned about optimal ways of measuring HRQL, and investigators may wish to see how different instruments perform. Aside from this sort of inquiry (which focuses on the instruments, rather than the intervention), an investigator may conclude that a single instrument will not yield all the relevant information. For example, utility and disease-specific measures contribute quite different sorts of data, and an investigator may want to use one of each.

Another, somewhat different, way of using multiple instruments is to administer a battery of specific instruments. One example of a clinical trial in which a battery of instruments were used to measure multiple aspects of HRQL is a double-blind, randomized trial of three anti-hypertensive agents in primary hypertension.[39] The investigators identified five dimensions of health they were measuring: the sense of well-being and satisfaction with life, the physical state, the emotional state, intellectual functioning, and ability to perform in social roles and the degree of satisfaction from those roles. Even within these five dimensions, additional components were identified. For example, separate measurements of sleep and sexual function were made. Patients taking one of the three drugs under investigation, captopril, scored better on measures of general well-being, work performance, and life satisfaction. The lesson for the clinician is clearly important: one can have an impact on not only the length, but also the quality of the patient's life according to choice of antihypertensive agent.

This approach, although comprehensive, has limitations. First, investigators must find a valid, responsive instrument for every attribute they wish to measure. Second, it is possible (indeed likely) that only some of the instruments chosen will show differences between the treatments under investigation. Unless one of the instruments has been designated as the primary measure of outcome before the trial started, different results in different measures may make interpretation difficult. The greater the number of instruments used, the greater the probability that one or more will favor one treatment or the other, even if the treatments' true effectiveness is identical. Thus, the alpha error (the probability of finding an apparent difference between treatments when in fact they their outcomes do not differ) increases with each new instrument used. Although this problem may be dealt with through statistical adjustment for the number of instruments used, such adjustment is seldom made.[40]

If only a small proportion of the instruments used favor an intervention (or if some measures favor the experimental treatment and other instruments favor the control) the clinician may be unsure how to interpret the results. For example, in a controlled trial in which patients with recent myocardial infarction were randomized to receive standard care, an exercise program, or a counselling program, Mayou and colleagues[41] rated many variables. These included work (change in physical activity, satisfaction, and time of return), leisure (change in physical activity and satisfaction, intensity, and exercise for health), marriage (change in protectiveness, discussion, and family), sex (change in frequency and satisfaction), satisfaction with outcome, compliance with advice, quality of leisure and work, psychiatric symptoms, cardiac symptoms, and general health. For almost all of these variables, there was no difference between the three groups. However, patients were more satisfied with exercise than with the other two regimens, families in the advice group were less protective, and the advice group had a greater number of work hours and frequency of sexual intercourse at follow-up after 18 months. We agree with Mayou's interpretation of the results: the study was viewed as not supporting the effectiveness of rehabilitation in improving HRQL. However, program advocates might argue that if even some of the ratings favored treatment, the intervention is worthwhile. The use of multiple instruments opens the door to such potential controversy.

A third problem with the battery approach arises if only one component or dimension of a multi-dimensional instrument is used. The validity of using only one section of an instrument is questionable. In general, the psychometric properties of the instrument will have been violated.

A final limitation of using a battery of instruments is that it gives no indication of the relative importance of various areas of dysfunction to the patient. For example, had Croog et. al. found that one antihypertensive agent disturbed sleep, while another had an adverse impact on sexual function, their approach would not have allowed determination of which drug had a greater net adverse impact on patients' lives.

CONCLUSIONS

A number of instruments for measuring quality of life in clinical trials are now available. Each instrument and study approach has its strengths and weaknesses; none is suitable for all situations. Furthermore, the relative merits of the different approaches requires further testing. Quality-of-life measurement may be particularly challenging in cross-national studies or studies involving children. Nevertheless, instruments which provide accurate, clinically important information are available for most health problems in which randomized trials are conducted. A variety of guides for selecting instruments are available.[42]

The state of the science is now such that investigators embarking on randomized trials should ask themselves if quality of life would be important to measure in their experiment. If the answer is yes, they should carefully consider the approach that would be optimal for their trial, and seek an instrument with established reproducibility, responsiveness, and validity.

REFERENCES

1. M. Bergner, Measurement of Health Status, *Med Care*. 23:696-704 (1985).
2. G. P. Prigatano, E. C. Wright, and D. Levin, Quality of life and Its Predictors in Patients With Mild Hypoxemia and Chronic Obstructive Pulmonary Disease, *Arch Intern Med*. 144:1613-1619 (1984).
3. G. H. Guyatt, M. Townsend, L. B. Berman, and S. O. Pugsley, Quality of life in Patients With Chronic Airflow Limitation, *Br J Dis Chest*. 81: 45-54 (1987).
4. E. Nelson, B. Conger, R. Douglass, and et. al., Functional Health Status Levels of Primary Care Patients, *JAMA*. 249:3331-3338 (1983).
5. J. Siegrist, Impaired Quality of life as a Risk Factor in Cardiovascular Disease, *J Chron Dis*. 40:571-578 (1987).
6. G. H. Guyatt, M. Townsend, S. O. Pugsley, and et. al., Bronchodilators in Chronic Airflow Limitation, Effects on Airway Function, Exercise Capacity and Quality of life, *Am Rev Respir Dis*. 135:1069-1074 (1987).
7. C. D. Toevs, R. M. Kaplan, and C. J. Atkins, The Costs and Effects of Behavioral Programs in Chronic Obstructive Pulmonary Disease, *Med Care*. 22:1088-1100 (1984).
8. R. A. Deyo, A. K. Diehl, and M. Rosenthal, How Many Days of Bed Rest for Acute Low Back Pain? A Randomized Clinical Trial, *N Engl J Med*. 315:1064-1070 (1986).
9. A. E. Fletcher, B. M. Hunt, and C. J. Bulpitt, Evaluation of Quality of life in Clinical Trials of Cardiovascular Disease. *J Chron Dis*. 40:557-566 (1987).
10. R. M. Kaplan, Quality of life Measurement, Measurement Strategies, *Health Psychol*. 115-116 (1985).
11. R. M. Kaplan, and J. W. Bush, Health-Related Quality of life Measurement for Evaluation Research and Policy Analysis, *Health Psychol*. 1:61-80 (1982).
12. G. W. Torrance, Measurement of Health State Utilities for Economic Appraisal, *Health Econ*. 5:1-30 (1986).
13. W. O. Spitzer, State of Science 1986: Quality of life and Functional Status as Target Variables for Research, *J Chron Dis*. 40:465-471 (1987).
14. R. A. Deyo, Measuring functional outcomes in therapeutic trials for chronic disease, *Controlled Clin Trials*. 5:223-240 (1984).
15. R. M. Kaplan, J. W. Bush, and C. C. Berry, Health Status: types of validity and the index of well-being, *Health Serv Res*. 11:478-507 (1976).
16. B. Kirshner, and G. H. Guyatt, A Methodologic Framework for Assessing Health Indices. *J Chron Dis*. 38:27-36 (1985).
17. G. H. Guyatt, C. Bombardier, and P. X. Tugwell, Measuring Disease-Specific Quality of life in Clinical Trials, *CMAJ*. 134:889-895 (1987).
18. G. H. Guyatt, S. Walter, and G. Norman, Measuring Change Over Time: Assessing The Usefulness of Evaluative Instruments, *J Chron Dis*. 40:171-178 (1987).
19. M. Bergner, R. A. Bobbitt, W. B. Carter, and B. S. Gilson, The Sickness Impact Profile: Development and Final Revision of a Health Status Measure, *Med Care*. 19:787-805 (1981).
20. C. R. Ott, E. S. Sivarajan, K. M. Newton, and et. al., A controlled randomized study of early cardiac rehabilitation: The Sickness Impact Profile as an assessment tool, *Heart Lung*. 12:162-170 (1983).

21. M. H. Liang, M. G. Larson, K. E. Cullen, and J. A. Schwartz, Comparative Measurement Efficiency and Sensitivity of Five Health Status Instruments for Arthritis Research, *Arthritis Rheum.* 28:542-547 (1985).

22. S. M. Hunt, S. P. McKenna, J. McEwen, E. M. Backett, J. Williams, and E. Papp, A quantitative approach to perceived health status: a validation study, *J Epidemiol Community Health.* 34:281-286 (1980).

23. D. L. Sackett, L. W. Chambers, A. S. MacPherson, C. H. Goldsmith, and R. G. McAuley, The Development and Application of Indices of Health: General Methods and a Summary of Results, *AJPH.* 67:423-428 (1977).

24. J. E. Ware, R. H. Brook, A. Davies-Avery, and et. al., "Conceptualization and measurement of health for adults in the health insurance study: Volume 1, Model of health and methodology," Rand Corporation, Santa Monica, CA, (1980).

25. C. R. MacKenzie, M. E. Charlson, D. Digioia, and K. Kelley, Can the Sickness Impact Profile Measure Change? An Example of Scale Assessment, *J Chron Dis.* 39:429-438 (1986).

26. R. A. Deyo, and R. M. Centor. Assessing the responsiveness of functional scales to clinical change: an analogy to diagnostic test performance. *J Chron Dis.* 39:897-906 (1986).

27. P. H. Sugarbaker, I. Barofsky, S. A. Rosenberg, and F. J. Gianola, Quality of life assessment of patients in extremity sarcoma clinical trials, *Surgery.* 91:17-23 (1982).

28. H. J. Sutherland, V. Dunn, and N. F. Boyd, Measurement of Values for States of Health with Linear Analog Scales, *Med Decis Making.* 3:477-487 (1983).

29. H. Llewellyn-Thomas, H. J. Sutherland, R. Tibshirani, and et. al., The measurement of patients' values in medicine, *Med Decis Making.* 449-462 (1982).

30. C. Bombardier, J. Ware, and I. J. Russel, Auranofin Therapy and Quality of life in Patients with Rheumatoid Arthritis; Results of a Multicenter Trial, *Am J Med.* 81:565-578 (1986).

31. G. H. Guyatt, L. B. Berman, M. Townsend, S. O. Pugsley, and L. W. Chambers, A Measure of Quality of life for Clinical Trials in Chronic Lung Disease, *Thorax.* 42:773-778 (1987).

32. G. Olsson, J. Lubsen, Es G. Van, and N. Rehnqvist, Quality of life after myocardial infarction: effect of long term metoprolol on mortality and morbidity, *Br Med J.* 292:1491-1493 (1986).

33. D. A. Mahler, D. H. Weinberg, C. K. Wells, and A. R. Feinstein, The Measurement of Dyspnea. Contents, interobserver agreement, and physiologic correlates of two new clinical indexes, *Chest.* 85:751-758 (1984).

34. R. F. Meenan, J. J. Anderson, L. E. Kazis, and et. al., Outcome Assessment in Clinical Trials. *Arthritis Rheum.* 27:1344-1352 (1984).

35. J. F. Fries, P. Spitz, R. G. Kraines, and H. R. Holman, Measurement of Patient Outcome in Arthritis, *Arthritis Rheum.* 23:137-145 (1980).

36. W. O. Spitzer, A. J. Dobson, J. Hall, and et. al., Measuring the quality of life of cancer patients, *J Chron Dis.* 34:585-597 (1981).

37. H. Schipper, J. Clinch, A. McMurray, and M. Levitt, Measuring the Quality of life of Cancer Patients: The Functional Living Index-Cancer: Development and Validation, *J Clin Oncol.* 2:472-483 (1984).

38. C. R. MacKenzie, and M. E. Charlson, Standards for the use of ordinal scales in clinical trials, *Br Med J.* 292:40-43 (1986).

39. S. H. Croog, S. Levine, M. A. Testa, and et. al., The Effects of Antihypertensive Therapy on the Quality of life, *N Engl J Med.* 314:1657-1664 (1986).

40. S. J. Pocock, M. D. Hughes, and R. J. Lee, Statistical problems in the reporting of clinical trials, *N Engl J Med.* 317:426-432 (1987).

41. R. Mayou, D. MacMahon, P. Sleight, and M. J. Florencio, Early Rehabilitation After Myocardial Infarction, *Lancet.* 2:1399-1401 (1981).

42. I. McDowell, and C. Newell, "Measuring Health: a guide to rating scales and questionnaires," Oxford University Press (1987).

EVALUATION OF BIAS AND VALIDATION OF SURVIVAL ESTIMATES IN A

LARGE COHORT OF AIDS PATIENTS TREATED WITH ZIDOVUDINE

Terri H. Creagh, M.S., M.S.P.H.

Clinical Manager
AIDS Research Consortium of Atlanta, Inc.
Atlanta, Georgia 30308

INTRODUCTION

As the epidemic of Acquired Immunodeficiency Syndrome (AIDS) has escalated over the last eight years, the need to find effective therapy has become increasingly more urgent. AIDS appears has a very high mortality rate, and the majority of the more than 30,000 reported deaths in the U.S. have occurred among persons less than 40 years old.[1] AIDS has become the most important health issue of our time, and the social and political issues surrounding the epidemic have been widely debated among all segments of society. The U.S. Food and Drug Administration (FDA) has relaxed its usual regulatory stance in an effort to allow possibly effective therapies to be made available to patients as quickly as possible. The urgency of the AIDS problem and the activism of patients has made virtually impossible the two double-blind placebo-controlled clinical trials normally required to demonstrate the efficacy and safety of a potential therapy. It has become clear that epidemiologic methods will become more and more important in validating and extending data obtained from traditional clinical trials. It is vital that we develop and validate these methods so that they can provide the most accurate assessment of the potential benefit of any therapeutic agent.

Zidovudine (AZT) was the first drug licensed by FDA for treatment of AIDS and advanced AIDS Related Complex (ARC). The approval was based on a single placebo-controlled clinical trial which demonstrated beneficial effects of therapy on survival of patients.[2] Subsequently, we employed epidemiologic methods to study zidovudine therapy in an open uncontrolled protocol involving 4,805 patients.[3] In the present work, we propose to critically examine this latter study for potential sources of bias, and to attempt to validate the original analysis in another study of patients being treated with zidovudine in 12 clinical sites throughout the United States.[4]

Results from the large open uncontrolled study of 4,805 patients showed the probability of survival 44 weeks after initiating therapy to be 73%. Survival was further enhanced in patients whose baseline hemoglobin was ≥ 120 g/l, whose baseline Karnofsky score (i.e., functional status) was $\geq 90\%$, and who began therapy within 90 days of diagnosis.[3] In studying the survival of patients treated with a common therapeutic agent, we must address the usual epidemiologic concerns, i.e., bias and differential loss to follow-up. The problems in defining a proper control group for such a cohort of treated patients are numerous. However, in collecting information on these patients treated with zidovudine under a Treatment IND program, we have attempted to further define the efficacy and safety of the drug while addressing some of the methodologic issues in analyzing data from the study. Thus, in seeking to validate the conclusions which may be drawn from such a study, we propose the following research questions:

Drug Epidemiology and Post-Marketing Surveillance, Edited by B.L. Strom
and G. Velo, Plenum Press, New York, 1992

1)   Can the direction and extent of the bias inherent in this uncontrolled trial be determined by examining and comparing subgroups in the cohort?

2)   Can the original survival estimates, which utilized censored observations, be validated in a sample from the original cohort in which the actual survival is known?

LITERATURE REVIEW

In 1981, a Los Angeles physician reported four cases of *Pneumocystis carinii* pneumonia (PCP) in previously healthy homosexual men.[5] The reports were baffling, because this type of pneumonia had previously been reported only in immunocompromised patients. Shortly after this initial report, other case studies of PCP and Kaposi's sarcoma in homosexual or bisexual men and intravenous drug users began to appear in the medical literature. Symptoms and signs included susceptibility to a number of opportunistic pathogens and malignancies, wasting, encephalopathy, severe immunodeficiency, persistent lymphadenopathy, unexplained fevers, and/or diarrhea. In addition, many patients developed thrombocytopenia, granulocytopenia, and/or progressive anemia. Symptomatic infected patients exhibited a marked reduction in CD4-positive (T4) lymphocytes and a decreased CD4/CD8 (T4/T8) ratio. This "syndrome" was also reported in patients who were hemophiliacs or who had previously received blood transfusions for other medical conditions. The picture of a disease transmitted by blood or body fluids quickly became apparent. A high incidence of this syndrome, initially called GRID (Gay-Related Immune Disorder), was also recognized in Haitians who had migrated to the United States. Transmission categories initially included Haiti as country of birth. It was later discovered that the Haitian connection to this epidemic had probably come by way of U.S. gay men vacationing in Haiti. In 1984, the discovery of a virus called lymphadenopathy virus (LAV) was reported by a group of researchers in France.[6] Shortly thereafter, an essentially identical virus isolated from Haitians in the United States was reported by a group of researchers at the National Institutes of Health.[7] It was later determined that these two viruses were essentially identical, and the virus was renamed the human immunodeficiency virus (HIV).[8] Once the virus was identified, development of a test for antibodies to the virus followed quickly. Testing of the blood supply in the United States began in 1984 and, currently, samples of all donated blood are tested for antibodies to HIV.

Although the initial transmission groups identified were gay/bisexual men, injecting drug users, hemophiliacs, blood transfusion recipients, and Haitians, it soon became apparent that the virus had no specific preference for any gender or group. It was clearly a virus transmitted by blood or body fluids, and thus by sexual intercourse or contact with infected blood. The virus began spreading into the heterosexual population through the injecting drug user (IDU) population, and infected children born to infected mothers began to appear.

As the epidemic began to widen, researchers recognized that the disease was rampant in certain parts of Africa.[9] In these countries, it appeared that the major mode of transmission was heterosexual intercourse. Additionally, it was known that needles used for injection are often reused in Africa because of shortages in medical supplies. This provides another potential route of infection.

A number of cohorts were established to investigate the epidemiology of HIV. The earliest and most well-known of these was a group of homosexual men for whom serum samples had been stored since the early 1970's for study of the spread of hepatitis B. A cohort of these patients was enrolled for continued prospective follow-up, and sera were analyzed retrospectively for the presence of antibody to HIV.[10] Through the study of the natural history cohorts and the epidemic in Africa and other countries outside the U.S., scientists were able to estimate that 270,000 cases of AIDS would occur in the United States by the end of 1991 and that up to 10 million people worldwide could be infected with HIV.[11] Public health implications were enormous. Major efforts were undertaken to provide education and funding for research to identify treatment and to better understand the etiology of this disease.

Many of the early drugs which were thought to have activity against the human immunodeficiency virus failed to show any clinical benefit. Among these were Suramin, HPA-23, AL-721, ribavirin and others.[12-15]

In 1985, scientists at the Wellcome Research Laboratories, in collaboration with colleagues at the National Cancer Institute (NCI), began screening a number of compounds for possible activity against HIV. In February, 1985, a compound was identified which appeared to have major activity against HIV.[16] Initially called azidothymidine, it is now known as zidovudine or AZT. In July, 1985, the first patient received zidovudine treatment in a Phase I clinical trial. The swiftness of approval by the Food and Drug Administration (FDA) to allow zidovudine to be tested in patients was a reflection of the urgency felt by the entire medical community for finding a solution to this problem. The Phase I trial studied the pharmacokinetics and bioavailability of zidovudine in AIDS patients and those with less advanced disease [i.e., AIDS-Related Complex (ARC)]. The study found that when the drug was administered orally, dose-independent kinetics were observed in the dose range of 2-10 mg/kg. The average bioavailability was 65% (range 52-75%). Although many of these early patients developed anemia and other milder adverse reactions, some apparent clinical benefits were noted. These included weight gain, increase in CD4-positive lymphocyte counts, and improvement in neurologic function.[17]

Because of these promising results, a Phase II, double-blind, placebo-controlled, clinical trial was initiated in February, 1986, to evaluate zidovudine as a treatment for AIDS patients who had a history of *Pneumocystis carinii* pneumonia (PCP) and for certain patients with advanced ARC. Patients were randomized to receive 250 mg of zidovudine or placebo every four hours around the clock. An independent Data and Safety Monitoring Board (DSMB) was convened to review the data periodically. After reviewing the data on 281 patients enrolled by September of 1986, the DSMB stopped the trial because of a dramatic difference in mortality in the two groups. At the time, 19 deaths had occurred in the placebo group while only one patient treated with zidovudine had died. Patients receiving zidovudine also experienced significantly fewer opportunistic infections compared to those receiving placebo. Additionally, zidovudine-treated patients showed improvements in performance status, weight gain, fewer and less severe symptoms associated with HIV disease, and an increase in CD4-positive lymphocyte counts when compared to placebo patients.[2] The most common adverse experiences seen in the drug-treated group were anemia and granulocytopenia, which tended to occur much more often in those patients whose pretreatment CD4 counts were 200/mm3 or less. Hematologic toxicity necessitated dose reduction or discontinuation in 34% of patients treated with zidovudine. Blood transfusions were administered to 31% of the drug-treated patients and 11% of the placebo patients.[18] Logistic regression analysis showed that predictors of hematologic toxicity were low CD4 count at study entry, low baseline hemoglobin, low baseline neutrophil count, and low baseline levels of vitamin B12. In addition, severe headache, nausea, insomnia, and myalgia were reported significantly more frequently in zidovudine-treated recipients compared to those receiving placebo.[18]

At the time the double-blind clinical trial was stopped, all patients were offered treatment with zidovudine. Follow-up of the trial cohort continued and survival was analyzed using the Kaplan-Meier method and intention-to-treat principles. Survival estimates for the original zidovudine-treated group were 84.5% and 41.2% after one and two years, respectively.[19] Both percentages were considerably higher than survival reported from contemporaneous natural history cohorts.[10]

When the trial ended, data were submitted to the Food and Drug Administration (FDA) as a New Drug Application (NDA) for zidovudine. During the six months required by the FDA to review these data, they permitted the institution of a Treatment Investigational New Drug (IND) program to provide zidovudine free of charge to any AIDS patient who had a history of PCP. Subsequently, 4804[*] patients were treated under this program before licensure for the drug was granted on May 19, 1987. Survival experience of these patients was followed and subsequently reported. Overall survival of the population was 73% at 44 weeks post-treatment initiation. However, in patients who began treatment with a hemoglobin of 12 or greater, a Karnofsky score of 90 or above, and who were within 90 days of AIDS diagnosis, survival at 44 weeks ranged from 85-90%.[3]

---

[*]Long-term follow-up revealed that one patient who was enrolled and was thought to have been treated actually never began treatment.

At the time of approval of the New Drug Application (NDA) for zidovudine, we initiated a new epidemiologic study which sought to monitor approximately 1000 patients treated with zidovudine in 12 U.S. sites under normal clinical practice. This study, called ZDV-502, involved abstraction of data from existing medical charts; it thus provided a means of evaluating the experience of patients being treated in "real-world" situations, i.e., outside the somewhat controlled environment of a clinical trial.[4]

MATERIALS AND METHODS

The original protocol for the zidovudine Treatment IND was approved by the Clinical Research Subpanel of the National Institute of Allergy and Infectious Disease (NIAID). Eligibility for enrollment was restricted to AIDS patients who had a histologically confirmed episode of PCP at any time in the past. Those who met specific entry criteria were eligible for enrollment between October 11, 1986, and March 24, 1987. Children, pregnant women, nursing mothers, and women of childbearing potential not employing barrier contraception or abstinence were excluded. Any licensed physician requesting enrollment of a patient meeting the protocol criteria was permitted to participate in this study. Patients were identified only by a study-specific 6-digit number. Confidentiality concerns precluded obtaining any patient names.

Criteria for patient enrollment in the Treatment IND included the following: a history of documented *Pneumocystis carinii* pneumonia (PCP); baseline hemoglobin ≥ 90 g/l; baseline granulocyte count $\geq 1000/mm3$; Karnofsky score ≥ 60 (changed to ">20" in the third month of the program); normal serum creatinine; platelet count $\geq 50,000$; AST not more than 3 times the upper limit of the normal range. [Enrollment required assessment of each patient's functional status using a standard grading system, the Karnofsky Score.[4] The score ranges from 0 (dead) to 100 (fully functional).]

Under the conditions of the protocol, all qualifying patients who gave informed consent were treated with open-label zidovudine. An initial dose of 200 mg every 4 hours was prescribed with the provision that the dose could be reduced for moderate hematologic toxicity, or therapy could be temporarily discontinued for severe toxicity.

Physicians completed monthly renewal forms while patients continued in the program. Certain data items, on these forms were required for continued drug shipments, e.g., laboratory data.

The protocol was open from October, 1986, to March, 1987. We employed a rigorous approach to data collection throughout the period. During that time, in addition to the required monthly prescription renewal forms, we provided a toll-free telephone number to physicians so they might supply information to a coordinating center or receive answers to questions concerning data or patient management. On the other hand, staff of the coordinating center used this telephone line to make literally thousands of telephone calls to physicians and pharmacists to clarify patient status or obtain missing data.

Near the end of the formal Treatment IND program, we mailed a short supplemental data form for each patient to his/her treating physician. We requested date and type of AIDS index diagnosis and absolute CD4+ lymphocyte cell count prior to zidovudine therapy. These supplemental forms were completed and returned for approximately 24% of enrolled patients. Where the date of AIDS diagnosis was different from the date originally supplied for confirmed PCP, we substituted the former date in the database. However, since only approximately 10% of the forms returned listed AIDS diagnosis dates greater than 30 days before the confirmed PCP date, it is likely that the use of the PCP date as an approximate date of AIDS diagnosis does not significantly affect the survival analysis. The only effect of using a post-diagnosis PCP date, in any case, would be to shorten survival estimates, as the AIDS diagnosis date, if different, could only be earlier than the PCP date.

The post-marketing survey strategy that began on May 1 involved two waves of mailed questionnaires in which we asked physicians to supply much of the same information they had supplied during the Treatment IND program, as well as some additional information. The principal difficulty, of course, was that after enrollment ended in March, the return of these forms became voluntary. However, we maintained the toll-free telephone number to both receive and transmit data. In addition, after the drug was licensed on March 19, 1987, and extending until September 15 of that year, we operated a limited drug distribution system because of limited drug supply. All patients filling a prescription for zidovudine were registered with a central coordinating center. This system provided computerized information on drug shipments. We could link patients who originally had been enrolled in the Treatment IND to specific drug shipments through their assigned patient number. Patients who continued to receive shipments were therefore assumed to be alive.

Patients were stratified into groups according to clinical status at the time of therapy initiation. Clinical status was measured principally by baseline hemoglobin, baseline Karnofsky score, and time since AIDS diagnosis (or confirmed PCP episode).

In November of 1987, we initiated a new intensive observational epidemiologic protocol (ZDV-502) to study patients being treated with zidovudine in normal clinical practice under the existing approved indications for the drug. We initiated this study in 12 clinical sites with the intent of monitoring approximately 1000 patients for two years. The study plan required that the records of all patients ever receiving zidovudine in these sites be screened as to their date of therapy initiation. We could therefore identify records of Treatment IND patients who were known to have been treated in those clinical sites, although they would not be enrolled in the new study. One benefit of this screening was to provide a means of estimating completeness of case ascertainment for the new epidemiologic study (ZDV-502). However, the validation of findings of the earlier Treatment IND analysis with data from a subcohort having more complete follow-up also became possible through this effort. The number of patients known to have been enrolled in the Treatment IND in the sites being monitored was determined by matching the physician of record with patient demographic characteristics and assigned Treatment IND numbers from the IND database. Patient names were not included in the data collected. The extent to which those IND patients were "found" through the screening process in those ZDV-502 sites was thought to approximate the extent of case ascertainment for the new epidemiologic study. Additionally, updated survival in the cohort of Treatment IND patients enrolled in these sites could be determined.

Records of all patients treated with zidovudine were screened by clinical monitors in each ZDV-502 site for unique Treatment IND number, date of birth, date on which zidovudine therapy was initiated, the last chart date on which patient-specific information was entered and the date and cause of death, if the patient had died. Where Treatment IND numbers were not available in the chart, but the date of therapy initiation indicated that the patient received therapy under the Treatment IND, a match was made according to patient demographic characteristics and birthdate with data from the Treatment IND database. By these criteria, a group of patients which should have been found by the study monitors was identified.

Medical records of a subcohort of 480 patients known to have been enrolled in the Treatment IND should have been available. Records of 322 patients were actually identified. We compared actual survival time to the estimates obtained from censoring the individual survival times at the last known date of follow-up during or following the Treatment IND program. This process provided a means of attempting to validate the survival estimates derived earlier from a life table analysis of the experience of the entire Treatment IND cohort.[3]

Patients who were "found" through the screening process were compared to patients who were "not found" by demographic characteristics and baseline clinical status to determine whether differences existed.

Analyses of baseline information for various patient categories were conducted using the Student-Newman-Keuls (SNK) Test option of the ANOVA procedure of the Statistical Analysis System (SAS), version 5.[20] The SNK test is a multiple-range procedure, but it essentially reduces to a t-test when comparisons are made between two groups.

Survival analyses employed the LIFETEST procedure of SAS[20] which computes nonparametric estimates of the survival distribution and generates life tables. LIFETEST calculates upper and lower confidence intervals according to the following formulae:

$$Upper = S + Z_{\alpha/2}V$$

$$Lower = S - Z_{\alpha/2}V$$

where S is the value of the survival function and V is the square root of the estimated variance.

Survival for patients not known to have died was measured from start of therapy until the last date on which information concerning clinical status was available. (Survival experience of those latter patients was "censored" at the date of last known clinical status.) Data were analyzed using an intention-to-treat approach. This method assumes that, for all treated patients, the intention was to continue to treat indefinitely. Survival is thus measured without regard to actual duration of therapy, and therefore the estimates obtained are conservative. The log rank statistic was used to compare the survival experience of various subcohorts of patients.

RESULTS

Examination of Bias. Four thousand eight hundred and four (4804) patients received zidovudine therapy under the Treatment IND program. Over 1,800 of these patients were enrolled during the first six weeks of the program. The remainder were enrolled over the succeeding 17 weeks. As shown in Table 1, the majority of patients were males (96.9%) and among these the primary AIDS transmission behavior was male-to-male sexual contact (87% of all patients). Many patients reported more than one AIDS risk behavior. Median age of the treated population was 36 years.

We can examine the problem of selection bias indirectly. Obviously, patients who had died prior to the beginning of this study could not be enrolled. There may therefore have been a tendency for patients who were enrolled to be "survivors." We attempted to examine the significance of this problem by examining a subcohort from a natural history cohort of the first 500 AIDS patients diagnosed in San Francisco. A group was identified from the San Francisco cohort diagnosed with PCP as the AIDS-defining opportunistic infection, excluding all those patients who died within the first 60 days after diagnosis (P. Bachetti and R. Chaisson, personal communication). We then selected patients in the open trial cohort who enrolled in the study within 60 days of the qualifying PCP episode or AIDS diagnosis, again excluding all those people who died within the first 60 days after diagnosis. We then had two subpopulations of "60-day survivors." These two groups, while not exactly equivalent, should be roughly comparable. Survival estimates at 11 months after diagnosis were 84.8% in the Treatment IND subcohort and 41.5% in the San Francisco subcohort. Survival at 18 months was 16.5% in the San Francisco group and 53.9% in the Treatment IND cohort.

The bias resulting from physicians having in some way selected patients for this study who may have had characteristics different from those who were not selected is a difficult one to analyze. We can approach this indirectly by comparing patients enrolled early in the study when physicians who were "AIDS experts" were the most likely to have participated to patients enrolled toward the end of the study when the participating physicians were likely to have been a much broader-based group. Table 2 shows a comparison of patients enrolled in the first six weeks to those enrolled during the final six weeks. It can be seen that, in the first six weeks, if anything, patients with more advanced disease were enrolling.

Information bias is also of some concern in regard to these data. Anecdotal reports have indicated that some physicians transfused anemic patients prior to enrollment in order that hemoglobin levels would be sufficient to qualify them for the study (i.e., > 90 g/l). This problem may be approached analytically by stratifying patients into various hemoglobin levels (Figure 1). While patients within the lowest hemoglobin stratum did have higher mortality, other strata showed progressively higher survival with higher baseline hemoglobin.

Similarly, when patients were stratified according to functional status, i.e., Karnofsky score, at the time of treatment initiation, survival time was positively correlated with baseline functional status (Figure 2).

Although losses to follow-up during the formal Treatment IND program were minimal (10%), these losses did increase after the formal IND period ended (March 24, 1987). Via telephone follow-up extending through June 30, however, 77% of patients were still being followed, even in the absence of any formal requirement for written

Table 1.   Description of Enrolled Population

	N	%
RISK CATEGORY:		
Male-to-Male Transmission	4167	86.7
I.V. Drug Abuser	287	6.0
Hemophiliac	65	1.4
Heterosexual	184	3.8
Transfusion Aquired	66	1.4
Other or Unknown	35	0.1
GENDER:		
Male	4657	96.9
Female	147	3.1
RACE:		
White, not Hispanic	3798	79.0
Black, not Hispanic	521	10.9
Hispanic	422	8.8
Pacific Islander, American Eskimo	21	0.4
American Indian	3	0.1
Other or Unknown	39	0.8

Table 2.   Comparison of Patients Enrolled During the First 6 Weeks of Treatment IND to Those Enrolled during Last 6 Weeks

	Enrolled in first 6 weeks N=1826		Enrolled in last 6 weeks N=937
% Male-to-Male Transmission	90.8%		82.3%[a]
% Male	97.4%	— N.S. —	96.1%
% White	84%		74.7%[a]
Median Baseline Hemoglobin	11.8	— N.S. —	11.8
Median Baseline Karnofsky Score	90	— N.S. —	90
Median Time-Since-PCP	139		59[b]
Median Age	36	— N.S. —	36

[a]p<.001 by chi-square
[b]p<.001 by Brown-Mood test for medians
N.S. = not significant

information. To examine the impact of the high loss-to-follow-up rate after June 30, several analyses were performed. First, patients lost to follow-up before July 1 were compared to those lost after June 30. Patients lost to follow-up early tended to have slightly more advanced disease at baseline (Table 3). Patients who were alive when the last known information was received on or before January 15, 1989, were compared to those known to have died. Those who subsequently died clearly had a poorer prognosis at the time of treatment initiation (Table 3).

As was reported elsewhere[3], survival data for which follow-up was most complete (through June 30) were compared with survival data available through September 15. For comparable time intervals, the survival estimates at each point up to 36 weeks were nearly identical (within two percentage points). The similarity of the estimates provide the rationale for reporting the later experience despite increasing losses to follow-up.

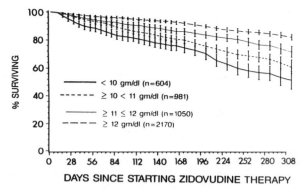

Figure 1.   Comparative Survival Experience by Hemoglobin Level at Therapy Initiation. Survival Curves with Confidence Limits.

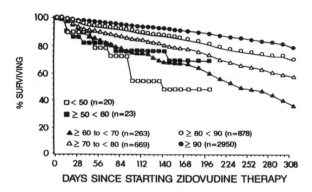

Figure 2.   Comparative Survival Experience by Karnofsky Scores at Therapy Initiation. Scores Range from 50 (Bedridden) to 100 (Healthy).

Validation Study. The validation study for these survival data was nested within our protocol ZVD-502. This involved an attempt to locate the records of 480 patients known to have been enrolled in 11 clinical sites during the Treatment IND. Patients who were "found" through the screening process were compared to patients who were "not found" by demographic characteristics and baseline clinical status to determine whether differences existed. Table 4 summarizes the new information we obtained on Treatment IND patients through the validation process. Among those patients who were known to be alive at the end of the Treatment IND and whose records were found, more than 70% were still alive at the time these records were reviewed. We obtained information beyond the end of September, 1987, on 62% of the patients not known to have died at that time. New information was obtained on over 50% of patients who had previously been withdrawn or lost to follow-up. Table 5 shows the expected and actual numbers of Treatment IND patients found through the screening process in each clinical site. In the 11 sites where screening had been completed, records of 480 Treatment IND patients should have been found through this process. This was approximately 10% of the total Treatment IND population. The actual number of these patients found was about 67% of the number known to have been enrolled in the Treatment IND in those clinical sites.

Table 6 shows the comparison of demographic characteristics of those patients "found" and those patients "not found" through the screening process. It can be seen that,

Table 3.   Characteristics of the Population by Survivorship and/or Follow-up Status (N=4804)

	Known Survivors (n=3033)				Patients Who Died (n=982)	Patients LFU[1] Before 7/1/87 (n=1246)				Patients LFU[1] After 6/30/87 (n=2579)
Age (Median)	36	—	N.S.	—	37	36	—	N.S.	—	36
% Male	97.2	—	N.S.	—	96.7	96.6	—	N.S.	—	97.1
% Male-to-Male Transmission	79.3	—	p<.02	—	74.3	75.5	—	p<.01	—	79.5
% Injecting Drug User (IDU)	7.4	—	N.S.	—	8.5	5.9	—	N.S.	—	7.2
% Hemophiliac	2.1	—	p<.001	—	1.5	1.6	—	p<.001	—	2.1
% Transfusion-aquired	3.0	—	p<.05	—	9.2	7.2	—	p<.01	—	3.5
% Heterosexually-aquired	2.5	—	p<.001	—	11.1	9.5	—	p<.001	—	3.2

[1]LFU=lost to follow-up
N.S.=not significant

Table 4.   Summary of New Patient Information Obtained through Validation Study

	Patient Status Determined Through Validation Study		
	No new information	Alive with additional follow-up	Known to have died
Patient Status at End of Formal Treatment IND Follow-up			
Known to have died (N=80)	80		
Known to be alive (N=23)	104 (44.9%)	91 (39.3%)	36 (15.9%)
Lost to follow-up (N=158)	78 (49.3%)	52 (32.9%)	28 (17.8%)
Withdrawn (N=11)	4 (36%)	3 (27%)	3 (27%)

Table 5.   Proportion of Records of Treatment IND Patients Found through Screening Process

Clinical Site	Proportion Found
B	100%
C	91.4%
E	64.3%
F	41.2%
G	70.8%
H	94.6%
I	75.0%
J	86.8%
K	50.0%
L	90.5%
M	25.0%
Overall Ascertainment	67.0%

as nearly as could be determined by the criteria available, no differences were apparent between those patients whose records were found and those not found. Table 7 shows a comparison of baseline clinical characteristics, i.e., clinical characteristics at the time therapy was initiated. Although the median Karnofsky scores and the elapsed time between diagnosis and start of treatment were comparable between those patients whose records were found and those not found, the median baseline hemoglobin was marginally lower among patients whose records were not located.

Tables 8 and 9 show these same comparisons using only those clinical sites in which case ascertainment was 85% or greater. We can see that the median baseline hemoglobin was slightly lower among the patients in these sites, the time between diagnosis and treatment was slightly longer, and patients were more likely to be male.

A cautious attempt to update survival requires that two analyses be made, i.e., a negative-bias case for the whole subcohort, assuming all the patients whose records were not found to have died, and a second analysis using data from those clinical sites where record ascertainment is at least 85% complete. Table 9 summarizes these findings. Although some slight differences were apparent on statistical analysis, it is doubtful that these differences were clinically relevant.

Survival data were available through 14 months post-treatment initiation in the most complete subset. It can been seen from the survival curve that survival in the larger cohort of "found" patients at 12 months post-therapy initiation was 73%. Survival post diagnosis was 90% at 12 months and 54% at 24 months. In the negative-bias case, which assumes each patient whose record was not found to have died 15 days after the last information was available, survival at 12 months after treatment initiation was 50%. (Table 10).

Survival at 12 months following PCP or other AIDS-defining diagnosis was 89% in our subcohort of patients from 5 Treatment IND sites with more complete record ascertainment and was 51% at 24 months. (Table 10). When we analyzed survival according to the predictive prognostic criteria which had emerged from the original survival analysis, the original reported trends were even more striking, i.e., patients whose pre-treatment hemoglobin level was higher, whose treatment began earlier after AIDS diagnosis, and whose functional status was good at the time of therapy initiation, showed a much higher survival rate than patients whose disease was more advanced at the time treatment was begun.

As a reference population, we can compare the reported 12-months survival in one of the major natural history cohorts which was closely contemporaneous with the Treatment IND cohort. Follow-up in this San Francisco natural history study is essentially complete for all patients. Survival at 12 months following diagnosis was reported to be 34.7% among AIDS patients diagnosed with PCP who survived at least 60 days beyond the date of diagnosis. Survival at 2 years in this cohort was 4.2% (Table 10).

DISCUSSION

We have attempted to validate a survival analysis of 4,804 AIDS patients treated with zidovudine. In so doing, we have attempted to identify and examine possible sources of bias. The variety of approaches to collection of data ensured that on June 30, i.e., three months after the end of Treatment IND patient enrollment, 77% of the original patient population were still being followed. This lends some credence to the validity of the data collected. However, we still have the same major concerns which apply to any epidemiologic study. These include selection bias, information bias, confounding, interaction, and differential loss to follow-up.

We compared patients who remained in the study for most or all of the observation period to those who were lost to follow-up sometime during the observation period. Those who remained in the study tended to be healthier, and therefore this bias was *away from the null*.

We compared patients who enrolled in the first 6 weeks of the study and thus contributed most to the later survival, to the patients enrolled during the final 6 weeks. Those patients enrolled very early tended to have more advanced disease and thus the direction of bias was *toward the null* (Table 2).

Table 6.   Demographics

	Total Population N=4804	Total Subcohort N=480	Records "Found" in Subcohort N=322				Records "Not Found" in Subcohort N=158
Median Age	36	36.4	36				39
% Male	96.9	99*	99.1	—	N.S.	—	98.7
% Male-to-Male Transmission	87.4	95.4**	94.7	—	N.S.	—	96.8
% IDU	6.0	1.9	2.5	—	N.S.	—	0.6
% Hemophiliac	1.4	0.2	0.3	—	N.S.	—	—
% Transfusion-acquired	1.4	0.2	0.3	—	N.S.	—	—
% Heterosexually-acquired	3.9	2.1	1.9	—	N.S.	—	2.5
% White	79.1	76.3	75.5	—	N.S.	—	77.9
% Black	10.8	13.5	13.0	—	N.S.	—	14.6
% Hispanic	8.8	8.8	9.6	—	N.S.	—	7.0

*p<.01 by Fisher's exact test
**p<.001 by chi-square
N.S.=not significant

Table 7.   Baseline Clinical Status

	Total Population (N=4804)				Total Subcohort (N=480)	Records "Found" In Subcohort (N=322)				Records "Not Found" In Subcohort (N=158)
Median Hemoglobin at Treatment Initiation	11.7	—	N.S.	—	11.9	12.1	—	p<.01*	—	11.4
Median Karnofsky Score at Treatment Initiation	90	—	N.S.	—	90	90	—	N.S.	—	90
Median Time since PCP or Other AIDS-Defining Diagnosis (Days)	100	—	N.S.	—	108.5	107	—	N.S.	—	120
% Known to Have Died	21.3	—	N.S.	—	20.4	34.3%	—	N.S.	—	35.4%
Median Follow-up (Days)	202	—	p<.001*	—	275	318	—	p<.001*	—	205

*by Brown-Mood test for medians

    Thus, the various biases which have been examined in studying the loss to follow-up in this cohort have been in opposing directions; therefore, the ultimate direction of the bias is unknown. However, the extent of bias in both directions was examined through estimates based on extreme assumptions. If all patients not known to have died were considered to be survivors throughout the study, 44-week survival would be 81% (95% C.I.=80.1 - 82.3%). If all patients who had been lost to follow-up were assumed to have died 15 days after the last report was received, 44-week survival would be 71% (95% C.I.=69.5 - 73.2%). The survival curve estimated from the actual database is somewhere between these two extremes. Even, in the "worst case" the survival is better than that seen in the San Francisco natural history cohort (Table 10). This gives some support to the idea that there is evidence of continued drug benefit in these data.

    Information bias is another concern in these data. One possible question is whether physicians complied with the requirement that patients enrolled in this study must have had a pathologically confirmed episode of *Pneumocystis carinii* pneumonia. The protocol required that physicians submit a signed copy of a pathology report which indicated that the patient's *Pneumocystis* was histologically confirmed. While it is believed that there were cases where these reports were simply photocopied and

Table 8.   Demographics

	Sites with More Complete Record Ascertainment N=158	All Other IND Patients N=4646
Median Age	36	36
% Male	99.1	96.8*
% Male-to-Male Transmission	92.6	87.1
% IVDA	4.2	6.1
% Hemophiliac	0.5	1.4
% Transfusion-acquired	0	1.5
% Heterosexually-acquired	2.8	3.9
% White	71.9	79.4
% Black	14.8	10.7
% Hispanic	10.6	8.7

*p=.03 (Fisher's exact test)

Table 9.   Clinical Status

	Sites with More Complete Record Ascertainment N=217		All Other IND Patients N=4587
Median Hemoglobin at Treatment Initiation	11.9	— p = .03* —	11.7
Median Karnofsky Score at Treatment Initiation	90		90
Median Time since PCP or Other AIDS-Defining Diagnosis (Days)	117	— p = .04* —	99
% Known to have Died	34.6%		20.7
Median Follow-up (Days)	260	— p = .001* —	199

*by Brown-Mood test for medians

submitted for multiple patients, we do not believe this practice was widespread. A close examination of these forms revealed that the vast majority of physicians did have the original reporting pathologist sign a copy of the pathology report and did submit that report as proof that the patient had PCP.

Reports indicated that some physicians chose to transfuse patients in order to increase their hemoglobin to required levels for enrollment. When patients were stratified according to hemoglobin level at the time of treatment initiation, a clear positive correlation emerged between baseline hemoglobin and survival time. (Figure 1). It is likely that baseline hemoglobin levels above 100 g/l were reliable, and thus survival in these patients can probably be considered to accurately reflect the data.

Since Karnofsky score is a subjective measure of functional status, it is possible that some physicians arbitrarily selected a score which would have qualified patients for the study. This may have been due, in part, to the fact that some physicians were not familiar with the Karnofsky scoring system. It is possible, however, that some physicians had patients who they believed could benefit from treatment, and that Karnofsky scores were adjusted accordingly. However, data indicate that patients with very low Karnofsky scores were not enrolled, i.e., patients who just barely met the Karnofsky score requirements numbered only 45 despite the fact that scores of >20 were permitted after

Table 10.

	% Surviving at 12 months after PCP or other AIDS-defining diagnosis (Negative Bias Case)[*]	% Surviving at 12 months after AZT initiation (Negative Bias Case)[*]
Population of Treatment IND Patients (N=4804)	85%	—
Subcohort of Treatment IND Patients (N=480)	87% (74%)	69% (50%)
Records "Found" in Subcohort (N=322)	90%[a]	73%
Records "Not Found" in Subcohort (N=158)	77%	48%
Population of IND Patients in 5 clinical sites with >85% case ascertainment	89%[b]	66%
Reference Population: Population of First 500 AIDS Patients in San Francisco-60 day survivors	34.7%[c]	—

[*] Negative Bias Case assumes each patient whose record was not found died 15 days after the last available information was obtained
[a] 54% at 2 years
[b] 51% at 2 years
[c] 4.2% at 2 years (P. Bachetti and R. Chaisson-personal communication)

January 1 (Figure 2). This would imply that adjusting the Karnofsky score to fit study criteria was not a widespread practice.

The approach to the problem of confounding in these data is a complex one. This was not the standard type of observational cohort study, since intervention was involved and no direct parallel control group was identified. However, since the study is clearly not a clinical trial in the sense of the "gold standard," the approach must be to treat it as an observational study. In this case, outcome is not progression to disease but is survival or non-survival of the patients. Therefore, potential confounders must be predictors of mortality or early mortality in patients and must be related to whatever exposure is being examined in the populations from which these patients are drawn. A number of potential confounders, as well as potential effect modifiers, were examined in these data. These included age, gender, race, transmission group, time-since-PCP (or other AIDS index diagnosis), baseline hemoglobin, and baseline Karnofsky score. Each of these covariates may also be considered as exposures in assessing confounding. Briefly, while gender, race, and risk category showed no statistically significant differences in survival among subgroups, time-since-PCP, baseline hemoglobin and baseline Karnofsky score were clearly positively correlated with survival. It is possible that confounding by disease status could have accounted for the findings. In the absence of an untreated concurrent comparison group, the independent effects of the variables which serve as surrogate markers for disease progression cannot be examined. However, because of the large disparity between survival estimates in this study and survival in similar groups in natural history cohorts, it is unlikely that these factors accounted for all the differences. It must be clear, however, that we can make inferences, however tenuous, only about a sample population which is predominately male with a history of male-to-male sexual exposure, but whose clinical stage of disease is reasonably comparable to the larger population of AIDS patients with a prior history of PCP.

Finally, we were able to validate the actual survival in a subcohort of approximately 7% of the original Treatment IND population. A comparison of those patient records which were located to those not located indicated that patients whose records were not found tended to have had a poorer baseline clinical status. Failure to include these patients' records in the data might create bias in two opposing directions: 1) patients who were sicker may have been more likely to have died or been lost to follow-up, thus biasing toward higher survival among those patients whose records were found, and 2) since it is known that patients with poorer bone marrow reserve cannot tolerate zidovudine as well as those with healthier marrow, patients who began therapy with lower hemoglobin may not have been able to take the drug long enough for beneficial effects to be manifested. Additionally, in sites where no automated records of zidovudine prescription were available, a mention in the chart of a very short course of the drug might have been missed in the screening process.

In conducting epidemiologic studies, it is important to draw samples which are representative of the population about which inferences are to be made. Thus, we should know whether the sample of all Treatment IND patients in these 11 clinical sites is a microcosm of the entire Treatment IND population of 4,804 patients. We examined data from those 5 clinical sites where patient record ascertainment was 85% or greater. When we compared the baseline clinical status of the 217 patients in these 5 sites to baseline clinical status of all other patients, the former group appeared to have had slightly more advanced disease. Therefore, the survival estimates we calculated for patients in the 5 sites are likely to be conservative. This leads us to conclude that we have not overestimated the survival experience of our cohort. The updated survival experience indicates that benefits of treatment continue to be apparent in this population. When the actual survival in patients from the 5 sites with good ascertainment was compared to the original survival estimates for the entire treated population, the survival curves were virtually superimposable.

Using the zidovudine program as a prototype, FDA has formulated fast-track approval procedures for drugs for life-threatening illnesses. The process involves short, limited preclinical and Phase II studies. The result of these new regulations is that sponsors of potential new AIDS therapies must be willing to essentially "put all their eggs in one basket." They will have to be willing to sponsor larger, more expensive Phase II trials with an "all or none" outcome. When Phase II results are positive, postmarketing pharmacoepidemiologic studies will take on increasing importance as they must now provide supporting data for therapeutic efficacy as well as safety.

In conclusion, because of the urgency of the AIDS crisis, it is clear that methods other than the "gold standard" double-blind placebo-controlled clinical trial must be employed to supplement clinical trial data. We report methods of validating well-designed epidemiologic studies. Through these methods, analysis of a subcohort of approximately 7% of the original 4,804 patients treated under the zidovudine Treatment IND has indicated that our initial assessment of the survival experience was correct. In the process of validation, additional data were obtained which extend survival estimates beyond one year after therapy initiation and show that survival is higher than would be expected from similar cohorts of untreated patients. Good epidemiological studies with careful validation and analyses of sources of bias can provide valuable data as we attempt to find more effective ways to use current therapies and to discover new therapies to combat this devastating pandemic.

REFERENCES

1.   HIV/AIDS Surveillance, Centers for Disease Control, October (1990).
2.   M. A. Fischl, D. D. Richman, M. H. Grieco, and et. al., The efficacy of azidothymidine (AZT) in the treatment of patients with AIDS and AIDS-related complex, *N Engl J Med.* 317:185-91 (1987).
3.   T. Creagh-Kirk, P. Doi, E. Andrews, and et. al., Survival experience among patients with AIDS receiving zidovudine, *JAMA.* 260:3009-3015 (1988).
4.   R. Moore, T. Creagh-Kirk, J. Keruly, et. al., Long-term safety and therapeutic response in patients treated with zidovudine (abstract), *J Clin Res Pharmacoepidemiol.* 4:130 (1990).
5.   M. Gottlieb, H. M. Schanker, P. T. Fan, and et. al., Pneumocystis pneumonia - Los Angeles, *MMWR.* 30:250-252 (1990).
6.   F. Barre-Sinoussi, C. Chermann, F. Rey, and et. al., Isolation of a T-lymphotropic retrovirus from a patient at risk for AIDS, *Science.* 220:868-870 (1983).
7.   R. C. Gallo, S. Z. Salahuddin, M. Popovic, and et. al., Frequent detection and isolation of cytopathic retroviruses (HTLV-III) from patients with AIDS and at risk for AIDS, *Science.* 224:500-503 (1984).

8.   J. Coffin, A. Haase and J. Levy. What to call the AIDS virus?, *N Engl J Med.* 319:492-497 (1984).

9.   N. Clumeck, J. Sonnet, H. Tallman, and et. al., AIDS in African patients, *N Engl J Med.* 319:492-497 (1984).

10. N. A. Hessol, G. W. Rutherford, A. R. Lifson, and et. al., The natural history of HIV infection in a cohort of homosexual and bisexual men: a decade of follow-up, 4th International Conf. on AIDS, Stockholm 4096, June (1988).

11. D. M. Barnes, Grim projections for AIDS epidemic, *Science.* 232:1589-1590 (1986).

12. B. D. Cheson, A. Levine, D. Mildvan, and et. al., Suramin therapy in AIDS and related diseases, Initial report of the U. S. suramin working group, *JAMA.* 258:1347-1351 (1987).

13. W. Rozenbaum, D. Dormont, B. Spire, and et. al., Antimoniotungstate (HPA 23) treatment of three patients with AIDS and one with prodrome (Letter), *Lancet.* 1:450-451 (1985).

14. P. S. Sarin, R. C. Gallo, D. I. Schneer, and et. al., Effects of a novel compound (AL 721) on HTLV-III infectivity in vitro, *N Engl J Med.* 313:1289-1290 (1985).

15. C. Crumpacker, W. Heagy, G. Bubley, and et. al., Ribavirin treatment of the acquired immunodeficiency syndrome (AIDS) and the acquired immunodeficiency syndrome related complex (ARC), *Ann Intern Med.* 107:664-674 (1987).

16. H. Mitsuya, K. J. Weinhold, P. A. Furman, and et. al., 3' azido-3'-deoxythymidine (BW A509U): an antiviral agent that inhibitis the infectivity and cytopathic effect of human T-lymphotropic virus HTLV-III/lymphadenopathy-associated virus in vitro, *Proc Natl Acad Sci USA.* 2:7096-7100 (1985).

17. R. Yarchoan, R. E. Klecker, K. J. Weinhold, and et. al., Administration of 3'-azido-3'-deoxythymidine, an inhibitor of HTLV-III/LAV replication, to patients with AIDS or AIDS-related complex, *Lancet.* 1:575-580 (1986).

18. D. D. Richman, M. A. Fischl, M. H. Grieco, and et. al., The toxicity of azidothymidine (AZT) in the treatment of patients with AIDS and AIDS-related complex, *New Engl J Med.* 317:192-197 (1987).

19. M. A. Fischl, D. D. Richman, D. M. Causey, and et. al., Prolonged zidovudine therapy in patients with AIDS and advanced AIDS-related complex, *JAMA.* 262:2405-2410 (1989).

20. SAS User's Guide: Statistics, version 5. Cary, NC, SAS Institute (1985).

THE TRIAZOLAM EXPERIENCE IN 1979 IN THE NETHERLANDS,

A PROBLEM OF SIGNAL GENERATION AND VERIFICATION

R. H. B. Meyboom, M.D.

Netherlands Centre for Monitoring of
Adverse Reactions to Drugs
Rijswijk, The Netherlands

INTRODUCTION

Triazolam (Halcion) was marketed as a hypnotic in the Netherlands early in 1978. There were tablets of three different strengths: 0.25, 0.5, and 1 mg. The product information recommended a dose of "0.25-0.5 mg for elderly patients who have not already been using a sedative or hypnotic drug and 0.5-1 mg for hospitalized patients, psychiatric patients, chronic alcoholics, and patients who were already using other hypnotic or sedative drugs" and included the advice to start in elderly and weakened patients with 0.25 mg. The paragraph on side effects read: "Sedation, hypotension, dizziness, impaired motor coordination, hiccup, headache or nausea are sometimes observed. These side effects usually occur when too high doses are taken."

Because of its short half-life, the drug was considered to have little residual effects and therefore to be comparatively free of side effects. Up to March 1979 only a small number of 14 reports concerning suspected adverse reactions to triazolam, used in various doses, had been received by the Netherlands Centre for Monitoring of Adverse Reactions to Drugs (NARD). These events included confusion, agitation, amnesia, twilight state, and unusual complaints such as globus feeling, "a burning tongue," "mucosal pain," or "painful eyes." Despite the small number, the reports attracted some attention because of their unusual nature.

THE 1979 EXPERIENCE

In April 1979 a Dutch psychiatrist, Van der Kroef, informed the NARD about four patients with psychotic disturbances which had developed in suspected connection with the use of triazolam, 0.5 or 1 mg. Leading symptoms were depersonalization, paranoid ideas, and -- remarkably -- perceptive changes with "hyperacusis," abnormal smell and numbness. Dr. Van der Kroef decided to present the experiences of his patients in the Netherlands Medical Journal. In the meantime, the NARD continued to receive small numbers of reports on suspected reactions to triazolam, again describing a variety of unusual symptoms, including a burning sensation of the skin, anorexia, taste loss, pain (head, neck, arm and hand), disorientation, derealization, aggression, amnesia, fears, nightmares, delirium, coma, and tremor after stopping. These reports came from family doctors and often contained only a brief description. As of July, when his article was published[1], Van der Kroef had in the meantime encountered a further 20 patients with possibly triazolam-associated psychic disturbances (his findings were later on summarized in the Lancet[2]), and he and some of his patients agreed to be interviewed on television. The subject was discussed on television on two more occasions and also the vice-chairman of the drug registration committee was interviewed, whereas another, rather sensational, interview with Van der Kroef appeared in a weekly magazine.

In the meantime more than a hundred new reports concerning triazolam were submitted to the NARD by many different physicians, often describing severe disturbances, and the NARD decided to send a letter to all physicians and pharmacists with information on the current situation and a request for the reporting of eventual additional experiences.[3] In this letter a list was included of apparently characteristic symptoms reported in association with triazolam; this list is reproduced in translation below:

> Depersonalization
> Derealization
> Paranoia
> Anxiety (periodically very strong), excitation, despair, suicidal inclination
> Aggressiveness
> Impulsive, inadequate behavior, sometimes twilight state; amnesia
> Hyperesthesia of sound, smell and taste
> Normal sounds reach intolerable intensity
> Numbness of limbs (acro-anesthesia), paresthesia
> Neck pain, headache (throbbing, very severe), cramps, often left-sided
> "Dysphagia": dry mouth, globus feeling, anorexia
> Nightmares, somnambulism
> Disorders of speech and writing
> After withdrawal: sweating, increased anxiety and need for sleep; longing to take triazolam again

The "Dear Doctor" letter was again followed by a large number of further reports of suspected adverse reactions to triazolam, often severe, and the Medicines Registration Committee subsequently suspended the license of the drug. Sensational publicity in the media on the one hand, and the disappearance of triazolam without much explanation by the authorities on the other, had somewhat confused the medical community, as was illustrated by the condemnation of the suspension of triazolam by Lasagna as a "trial by media"[4]. Lasagna, however, had not had access to the data reported to the NARD and was only incompletely informed. In fact there was, and still is, no evidence at all that the Medicines Registration Committee - which is a legal and non-political body - has been sensitive to public pressure. Nevertheless, the possible interference with the confidence of the medical profession emphasized the need for an extremely cautious assessment of the available evidence and the subsequent decision making.

THE DILEMMA

Following the suspension of the license of triazolam, the Drug Registration Committee had a maximum of six months for investigation and to decide upon the conditions for reintroduction of triazolam. At that moment the situation can be summarized as follows. On the one hand, the NARD had received approximately 1000 case reports on triazolam from about 600 different physicians, exceeding the number of reports on all other drugs together in 1979. These reports included a confusing multitude of symptoms, encompassing almost the entire field of psychiatry, and in many cases the relationship with triazolam was uncertain. Despite the complexity of the reactions, there were some indications of the existence of a "syndrome," including the following phenomena:

> Anxiety; fears
> Agitation; aggression
> "Dysesthesia" (i.e., hyperacusis, photophobia, paresthesia, dysgeusia, parosmia, pains)
> Depression
> Paranoid ideation
> Depersonalization & derealization
> Amnesia

160

In addition behavioral abnormalities, symptoms of the autonomous nervous system, and dependence were reported. Especially the frequently reported perceptual disturbances such as hyperacusis seemed to be a "red line" connecting the reports; these could on the other hand also be explained as signs of hysteria.

At that moment, when the Medicines Committee had to make a decision, there was more or less uncertainty with regard to the following questions:

1. Is the syndrome really existent and, if so, can it be caused by triazolam?
2. How frequent are these reactions?
3. Which mechanisms are involved?
4. Is triazolam different?
5. Why only in the Netherlands?

These uncertainties may have contributed to the failure of the Medicines Registration Committee and the Upjohn Company to agree on new terms for reintroduction of triazolam in the Netherlands. As a consequence, the suspension of the license had to be followed by a withdrawal. As will be discussed below, triazolam was not reregistered until 1990, 11 years later, in a different strength and with a considerably different data sheet.

TEN YEARS LATER

The purpose of the present review is to discuss these questions again, more than 10 years later, in the light of the body of knowledge which has in the meantime become available.

Is the Syndrome Really Existent and, if So, Can It Be Caused by Triazolam?

Until 1979 a complex of symptoms, as was reported with triazolam, was not a recognized syndrome and had not been described previously in association with triazolam or any other drug. Uncertainty in this respect continued until 1981, when a very similar cluster of symptoms, including the intriguing hyperacusis and other perceptual disturbances, was almost simultaneously described by Petursson and Lader[5,6] and Tyrer et al.[7,8] The list of the symptoms as presented by Petursson and Lader[5] is reproduced below:

Anxiety, tension
Agitation, restlessness
Bodily symptoms of anxiety
Irritability
Lack of energy
Impaired memory and concentration
Depersonalization, derealization
Sleep disturbance
Tremor, shakiness
Headache
Muscle pains, aches, twitchings
Loss of appetite
Nausea, dry retching
Depression
Perspiration
Metallic taste, hyperosmia
Blurred vision, sore eyes, photophobia
Incoordination, vertigo
Hyperacusis
Paraesthesia
Hypersensitivity to touch, pain
Paranoid reaction

Interestingly, the syndrome was not associated with triazolam, however, but with other, well known, benzodiazepines (i.e., diazepam and lorazepam) and had occurred in patients after stopping these drugs. These studies disclosed the existence of a specific (but previously not recognized) benzodiazepine witdrawal syndrome, which appeared to have much in common with the "triazolam syndrome" as reported in the Netherlands. Several other studies have since confirmed the existence of the benzodiazepine withdrawal syndrome. Especially the article of Ashton gave a comprehensive description of the very complex symptomatology of this syndrome[9]; she described almost the entire scale of psychic and bodily symptoms which had a few years earlier in association with triazolam caused so much confusion. Furthermore, she also referred to the occurrence of the syndrome during the use of benzodiazepines.

Can the first part of the question now be positively answered. A substantial number of case reports in the medical journals in several countries[10-27], have confirmed that triazolam can indeed cause serious psychic reactions, even in small doses.[19] In this respect the intelligent study of Bixler et al[20], comparing case reports concerning triazolam, temazepam, and flurazepam, as collected by the USA Food and Drug Administration, is especially of significance. Moreover, similar experiences have been reported in connection with other short acting benzodiazepine derivatives such as midazolam.[28,29]

In fact there have already, in an early stage, been some indications of a possible problem with triazolam. In 1976 Kales et. al. briefly reported on remarkable experiences in two patients.[32] One observation concerned a patient who during a night in the sleep laboratory (on 0.5 mg triazolam) had a biliary colic, caused considerable excitement in the laboratory. The next morning, however, she appeared to have a complete amnesia for the episode. The other patient was included in an outpatient study of triazolam. When entering the kitchen in the morning, she found a fully prepared breakfast table, which she had apparently prepared herself after she had taken triazolam and gone to bed, but again she had no memory thereof. Furthermore the Halcion product monograph as approved in Canada in 1978, already included a special warning for the occurrence of amnesia and listed a number of possible side effects, not mentioned in the data sheet in the Netherlands.

How Frequent Are These Reactions?

Once a new adverse reaction has been identified, it is usually very important to assess the frequency with which the reaction occurs. Unfortunately there is still uncertainty with regard to the frequencies of serious adverse reactions with different doses of triazolam. Several studies have reported only very small frequencies of adverse reactions.[33,34] Other studies have, on the other hand, revealed a different picture. In a small study on psychiatric patients, Soldatos et al, observed adverse effects in all five patients using 0.5 mg triazolam.[18] Adams and Oswald observed a reactive psychosis in two of 50 patients on triazolam (0.5 mg); seven patients had panic attacks and several others had additional side effects.[21] Although these differences are difficult to explain, several factors may have been involved. A connection between triazolam and a seemingly coincidental psychiatric illness may have been overlooked in some studies, or such patients may have withdrawn from the study without further explanation. Studies merely collecting "patient-nights" by short interviews of patients using triazolam for only short periods, may fail to detect adverse reactions even when large numbers of patients are involved. The side effects in the study of Soldatos et al were identified because the patients were cautiously investigated. Although the absolute frequency is still uncertain, the already mentioned study of Bixler et. al., suggests that serious adverse reactions are more frequent with triazolam as compared with the hypnotics temazepam and flurazepam.[20] Although adverse reactions have occurred already with low doses, it is reasonable to assume that reactions are more frequent and more severe when high doses are used.

Which Mechanisms and Factors Are Involved?

Although "paradoxical reactions" with excitation and aggression had occasionally been described with various benzodiazepines, many of the disturbances reported in association with triazolam could in 1979 not be explained in pharmacological terms.

Only symptoms such as sedation, confusion, depression, and amnesia were understandable as benzodiazepine effects. Since the doses used in the Netherlands were about two to four times higher than are nowadays used, it is not surprising that strong benzodiazepine-type side effects occurred. Since the discovery of the benzodiazepine withdrawal syndrome and its striking similarity to the triazolam reactions, especially with regard to the peculiar perceptive disturbances, it is reasonable to assume that withdrawal was an important mechanism involved. In other words, the triazolam syndrome can now be understood as a combination of strong benzodiazepine effects and withdrawal effects. The consequences of the half lives of different benzodiazepines with regard to effect and withdrawal, and of the rapidly alternating "on" and "off" states with triazolam, have been elucidated by Oswald.[35]

Although the benzodiazepine withdrawal syndrome is now well established, it probably does not occur in all users. Apparently there are people who are sensitive to the withdrawal of a benzodiazepine and others who are not. Although an exact figure is not known, a reasonable estimation is that about 30-45% of people are susceptible to benzodiazepine withdrawal[36] and, as is discussed below, some individuals may be especially vulnerable to drugs with a pharmacologic profile such as triazolam.

Is Triazolam Different?

Triazolam is undoubtedly a benzodiazepine derivative and has the corresponding pharmacological effects. Our knowledge of the physiology of benzodiazepine-receptors and of the diversity of the pharmacology of various benzodiazepines is still incomplete, however, and is likely to increase in the years to come; the latter may be especially true for drugs such as triazolam or alprazolam (which has also been associated with behavioral disturbances).[37-39] Although being a benzodiazepine, some features of triazolam may have far reaching consequences and practically distinguish it from "traditional" benzodiazepines.[40] Much of the experience with benzodiazepines, collected in the past few decades, referred to long acting drugs such as diazepam, chlordiazepoxide, or flurazepam. Triazolam had originally been advocated for its short duration of action and absence of residual effects. It is exactly for the same reason, however, why withdrawal may especially be a problem with this drug. The severity of a withdrawal reaction is influenced by the height of the dose in which the drug is used, the duration of use, and the rapidity of withdrawal (i.e., abrupt or gradual). Triazolam is a very potent drug and the doses used in 1979 were two to four times higher than those that are used nowadays. Used as a hypnotic triazolam is taken only once per 24 hours. With a half life in the range of only a few hours, withdrawal is very rapid and symptoms can already occur within the dosage interval[35], i.e., also in patients who continue to use the drug. Withdrawal effects have been observed with a small dose of only 0.125 mg triazolam[41], and already when triazolam was used for only a single night.[42] Withdrawal may become manifest as early morning awakening, increased day-time anxiety and rebound insomnia[43-47]; also more serious reactions may occur, including seizures[48] and delirium, as can be illustrated with a patient with an acute withdrawal psychosis after a single overdose of triazolam.[49] When triazolam withdrawal is abrupt and acute, it may apparently cause profound effects in susceptible people. Hypnotics such as flurazepam or nitrazepam, on the other hand, accumulate and produce a residual blood level around the clock. When the use of such a drug is discontinued, the blood level decreases only slowly and withdrawal symptoms are delayed and tempered.

Also in another respect triazolam is different. The onset of effect is very rapid, leaving the user little or no time to realize his or her altered state of conciousness. A user should ensure to take the tablet when already being safe in bed, or may otherwise later on awaken in the living-room, kitchen, or anywhere else.[14] Furthermore, the rapid and short action enables the administration of comparatively high doses of triazolam. After an overdose the individual will rapidly be in a state of profound intoxication, lasting for only a couple of hours. In this state he or she has strongly impaired mental functions and no memory, but may not be noticably "drunken." Because of amnesia the patient or victim exposed to triazolam has no recollection of anything which has happened (and may even remain unaware that something has happened at all). An equipotent dose of diazepam, on the other hand, would have caused noticable sedation of prolonged duration. Handwriting while under the influence of triazolam could not be distinguished graphologically from normal.[50] The criminal potentials of triazolam are frightening.

Also with regard to amnesia, triazolam is rather different as compared with traditional long acting benzodiazepine derivatives. With diazepam, for example, a therapeutic degree of amnesia (e.g., for minor surgery) usually requires the parenteral administration of a high dose, while triazolam easily causes amnesia already after oral use of a normal hypnotic dose.[51-56] Recent evidence shows that memory impairment caused by triazolam may (even unknowingly) persist after sedation has disappeared.[56] Perhaps effect and withrawal may occur at the same time.[21]

Triazolam-like psychic and behavioral disturbances have been observed with other strong and short acting benozodiazepines such as midazolam[22,23] but also with derivatives with a longer half life, e.g., lorazepam.[24,25] This is in support of the view that the pharmacokinetic properties may at least partly be responsible for the reactions as observed with triazolam.

Why Only in the Netherlands?

Differences in the occurrence of drug-related diseases in various countries are an intriguing aspect of pharmacoepidemiology. Why SMON, for example, has largely been restricted to Japan, has never been fully explained. While studying differences among countries, the first thing to do is to assess the consumption of the drug concerned in these countries. During the triazolam incident in 1979 in the Netherlands, similar problems were not reported in other countries. It was not immediately realized, however, that the Netherlands and Belgium had been the very first countries where triazolam was introduced. In July 1979 many other countries had also registered the drug, but only recently and the experience was still limited. In fact the majority of all triazolam tablets sold had been distributed in the Netherlands and Belgium. As has been discussed above, characteristic triazolam reactions have since been reported in many other countries and have recently also received attention of the public media in the USA[59] and Norway.[60] Increasing problems with triazolam, e.g., in West Germany[61], France[62], and the USA, have contributed to the world-wide withdrawal of 1 mg and later on also 0.5 mg triazolam tablets and of lowering of the recommended doses. In some other countries (e.g., in Denmark)[63], on the other hand, voluntary reporting does not seem to have detected a special problem with triazolam. Since underreporting of adverse reactions is extensive[64], especially when a reaction is not well known to practitioners, however, a voluntary reporting system has little value for providing proof of the safety of a drug.

SUMMARY

In 1979 the Netherlands Centre for Monitoring of Adverse Reactions to Drugs received a remarkably large number of reports of suspected adverse reactions to the new hypnotic triazolam, exceeding that of all other drugs together in the same year. Many of these, often serious, reports described an unusual complex of symptoms, including strange perceptive disorders such as hyperacusis, photophobia, and abnormal smell and taste. Although these suspected reactions could at that time not be understood as pharmacological effects and despite uncertainty with regard to the pathogenesis and frequency of these reactions, the license of triazolam was suspended and later on withdrawn.

Since then a specific benzodiazepine withdrawal syndrome has been unmasked, which is in many respects similar to the reactions reported with triazolam. International experience has in the past ten years confirmed that triazolam can cause serious psychic adverse reactions. These reactions can probably be explained as a combination of rapidly alternating strong benzodiazepine effects and withdrawal effects. The Netherlands and Belgium were the first countries in the world to approve triazolam. Since the introduction of triazolam in other countries, similar reactions have been reported in several of these countries. In recent years the recommended dose of triazolam has decreased considerably, and tablets with a strength of 1 mg and 0.5 mg, which were widely used in the Netherlands, have worldwide been withdrawn.

In retrospect the signal in the Netherlands has been an valuable early warning rightly casting doubt on the safety of triazolam and the original dose recommendations. It is still uncertain, however, with which frequencies serious adverse reactions occur with different doses of triazolam.

REFERENCES

1.   C. Van der Kroef, Halcion, een onschuldig slaapmiddel?, *Ned Tijdschr Geneesk.* 123:1160-1 (1979).
2.   C. Van der Kroef, Reactions to triazolam, *Lancet.* 2:526 (1979).
3.   R. H. B. Meyboom, Psychische stoornissen tijdens het gebruik van triazolam (Halcion), Letter to all physicians and pharmacists, 16 juli (1979).
4.   L. Lasagna, The Halcion story: trial by media, *Lancet.* 1:815-6 (1980).
5.   H. Petursson, and M. H. Lader, Withdrawal from long-term benzodiazepine treatment, *Brit Med J.* 283:643-5 (1981).
6.   M. Lader, and H. Petursson, Long-term effects of benzodiazepines, *Neuropharmacology.* 22:527-33 (1983).
7.   P. Tyrer, D. Rutherford, and T. Huggett, Benzodiazepine withdrawal symptoms and propranolol, *Lancet.* 1:520-22 (1981).
8.   P. Tyrer, and R. Owen, Gradual withdrawal of diazepam after long-term therapy, *Lancet.* 1:1402-6 (1983).
9.   H. Ashton, Benzodiazepine withdrawal: an unfinished story, *Brit Med J.* 288:1135-40 (1984).
10.   T. R. Einarson, Hallucinations form triazolam, *Drug Intell Clin Pharm.* 14:714-5 (1980).
11.   T. R. Einarson, and E. S. Yoder, Triazolam psychosis, *Drug Intell Clin Pharm.* 16:330 (1982).
12.   B. Trappler, T. Bezeredi, Triazolam intoxication, *Can Med Assoc J.* 126:893-4 (1982).
13.   A. N. Singh, Chemij, and J. Jewell, Treatment of triazolam dependence with a tapering withdrawal regimen, *Can Med Assoc J.* 134:243-5 (1986).
14.   J. W. Mostert, Die Halcion-affere, *S Afr Med J.* 59:967 (1981).
15.   R. Poitras, A propos d'épisodes d'amnésies antérogrades associés a l'utilisation du triazolam, *L'Union Med Canada.* 109:427-29 (1980).
16.   T. L. Tan, E. O. Bixler, A. Kales, R. J. Cadieux, and A. L. Goodman, Early morning insomnia, daytime anxiety, and organic mental disorder associated with triazolam, *J Family Practice.* 20:592-4 (1985).
17.   Q. R. Regestein, and P. Reich, Agitation observed during treatment with newer hypnotic drugs, *J Clin Psychiatry.* 46:280-3 (1985).
18.   C. R. Soldatos, P. N. Sakkas, J. D. Bergiannaki, and C. N. Stefanis, Behavioural side effects of triazolam in psychiatric inpatients: report of five cases, *Drug Intell Clin Pharmac.* 20:294-7 (1986).
19.   J. F. Patterson, Triazolam syndrome in the elderly, *South Med J* 80:1425-6 (1987).
20.   E. O. Bixler, A. Kales, B. H. Brubaker, and J. D. Kales, Adverse reactions to benzodiazepine hypnotics: spontaneous reporting system, *Pharmacology.* 35:286-300 (1987).
21.   K. Adam and I. Oswald, Triazolam 0,5 mg as an hypnotic causes daytime anxiety.
22.   J. B. Weilburg, G. Sachs, and W. E. Falk, Triazolam-induced brief episodes of secundary mania in a depressed patient, *J Clin Psych.* 48:492-3 (1987).
23.   R. Denson, Involuntary self-intoxication with triazolam, *Psych J Univ Ottawa.* 12:242-3 (1987).
24.   J. A. E. Flemming, Triazolam abuse, *Can Med Assoc J.* 129:324-5 (1983).
25.   E. J. Lynn, Triazolam addiction, *Hosp Community Psychiatry* 36:779-80 (1985).
26.   J. A. Flemming, K. Rungta, and T. Isomura, Withdrawal regimen for triazolam-dependent patients, *Can Med Assoc J* 134:1230-1 (1986).
27.   K. R. Olson, L. Yin, J. Osterloh, and A. Tani, Coma caused by trivial triazolam overdose, *Am J Emerg Med.* 3:210-1 (1985).
28.   D. Schneider-Helmert, Dämmerzustände nach dem Hypnotikum Midazolam, *Schweiz med Wschr* 115:247-9 (1985).
29.   M. Häcki, Amnestische Episoden nach einnahme des Hypnotikums Midazolam, Wirkung oder Nebenwirkung?, *Schweiz med Wochenschr.* 116:42-4 (1986).
30.   B. Poyen, R. Rodor, Jouve-Bestagne, M. C. Galland, R. Lots, and J. Jouglar, Amnésie et troubles comportemantaux d'apparence délictuelle survenus apres ingestion de benzodiazépines, *Thérapie* 37:675-8 (1982).

31. J. L. Fouilladieu, J. d'Enfert, M. Zerbib, N. Yegaheg, F. Baudin, and C. Conseiller, Troubles comportementaux secondaires a la prise de benzodiazépines, *Presse Méd* 14:1009-12 (1985).

32. A. Kales, J. D. Kales, E. O. Bixler, M. B. Scharf, and E. Russek, Hypnotic efficacy of triazolam: sleep laboratory evaluation of intermediate-term effectiveness, *J Clin Pharmacol* 16:399-406 (1976).

33. N. Macleod, Triazolam: monitored release in the United Kingdom, *Brit J Clin Pharmacol*. 11:51S-53S (1981).

34. A. N. Singh, and B. Saxena, Double-blind cross-over comparison of triazolam and flurazepam in hospitalized psychiatic patients with insomnia, *Curr Ther Res Clin Exp*. 27:627-34 (1980).

35. I. Oswald, Criteria for selecting an hypnotic, TGO tijdschrift voor Therapie, *Journal for Drugtherapy and Research*. 9:480-6 (1984).

36. H. Ashton, Risk of dependence on benodiazepine drugs: a major problem of long term treatment, *Brit Med J*. 298:103-4 (1989).

37. J. F. Rosenbaum, S. W. Woods, J. E. Groves, and G. L. Klerman, Emergence of hostility during alprazolam treatment, *Am J Psychiatry*. 141:792-3 (1984).

38. D. L. Gardner, and R. W. Cowdry, Alprazolam-induced dyscontrol in borderline personality disorder, *Am J Psychiatry*. 142:98-100 (1985).

39. A. Strahan, J. Rosenthal, M. Kaswan, and A. Winston, Three case reports of acute paroxysmal excitement associated with alprazolam treatment, *Am J Psychiatry* 142:859-61 (1985).

40. A. Kales, Benzodiazepine hypnotics and insomnia, *Hosp Pract (Off)* 25:Suppl 3,7-21, discussion 22-3 (1990).

41. A. J. Bayer, E. M. Bayer, M. S. J. Pathy, and M. J. Stoker, A double-blind controlled study of chlormethiazole and triazolam as hypnotic in the elderly, *Acta Psychiatr Scand* 73, suppl 329:104-11 (1986).

42. M. Mamelak, A. Csima, and V. Price, The effect of a single night's dosing with triazolam on sleep the following night, *J Clin Pharmacol*. 30:549-55 (1990).

43. K. Morgan, and I. Oswald, Anxiety caused by a short-life hypnotic, *Brit Med J*. 284:942 (1982).

44. A. Kales, C. R. Soldatos, E. O. Bixler, and J, D. Kales, Early morning insomnia with rapidly eliminatied benzodiazepines, *Science*. 220:95-7 (1983).

45. A. Kales, and J. D. Kales, Sleep laboratory studies of hypnotic drugs: efficacy and withdrawal effects, *J Clin Psychopharmacol*. 3:140-50 (1983).

46. C. A. L. Moon, S. I. Ankier, and G. Hayes, Early morning insomnia and daytime anxiety - a multicentre general practice study comparing loprazolam and triazolam, *Brit J Clin Practice*. 39:352-8 (1985).

47. R. Fontaine, G. Chouinard, and L. Annable, Rebound anxiety in anxious patients after abrupt withdrawal of benzodiazepine treatment, *Am J Psychiatry*. 141:848-852 (1984).

48. A. Y. Tien, and K. Gujavarty, Seizure following withdrawal form triazolam. *Am J Psychiatry*. 142:1516-7 (1985).

49. A. J. Heritch, R. Capwell, and P. P. Roy-Byrne, A case of psychosis and delirium following withdrawal from triazolam, *J Clin Psychiatry*. 48:168-9 (1987).

50. D. E. Boatwright, Triazolam, handwriting, and amnestic states: two cases, *J Forensic Sci*. 32:1118-24 (1987).

51. R. J. Shader, and D. J. Greenblatt, Triazolam and anterograde amnesia: all is not well in the z-zone, *J Clin Pharmacol*. 3:273 (1983).

52. T. Roth, K. M. Hartse, P. G. Saab, P. M. Piccione, and M. Kramer, The effects of flurazepam, lorazepam, and triazolam on sleep and memory, *Psychopharmacology*. 70:231-7 (1980).

53. M. B. Scharf, K. Fletcher, and J. P. Graham, Comparative amnestic effects of benzodiazepine hypnotic agents, *J Clin Psychiatry*. 49:134-7 (1988).

54. H. H. Morris, and M. L. Estes, Traveler's amnesia, transient global amnesia secondary to triazolam, *JAMA*. 258:945-6 (1987).

55. J. A. Ewing, W. J. Elliott, H. B. Radack, H. H. Morris, M. L. Estes, and M. Cohen, You don't have to be a neuroscientist to forget everything with triazolam, but it helps, *JAMA*. 259:350-2 (1988).

56. M. B. Scharf, R. Kauffman, L. Brown, J. J. Segal, and J. Hirschowitz, Morning amnestic effects of triazolam, *Hillside J Clinical Psychiatry*. 38-45 (1986).
57. A. Kales, C. R. Soldatos, E. O. Bixler, and J. D. Kales, Rebound insomnia and rebound anxiety: a review, *Pharmacology*. 26:121-37 (1983).
58. A. Kales, E. O. Bixler, A. Vela-Buena, C. R. Soldatos, D. E. Niklaus, and R. L. Manfredi, Comparison of short and long half-life benzodiazepine hypnotics: triazolam and quazepam, *Clin Pharmacol Therap*. 40:378-86 (1986).
59. C. Ehrlich, California, September, 60-67 (1988).
60. G. Gadeholt, and O. Brørs, Tilvaerelsen med og uten Halcion, *Tidsskr Nor Laegeforen* 110:878 (1990).
61. Arznei-Schnellinformationen, Halcion 0,5 mg Tabletten: Verzicht auf Zulassung; Halcion 0,25 mg Tabletten: Aenderung der Packungsbeilage, *Bundesgesundhbl*. 31:107 (1988).
62. Halcion 0.5 mg suspended in France, Scrip No 1189, 24, 20 maart (1987).
63. J. S. Schou, Triazolam: adverse effectsin relation to dosage, *Pharmacol Toxicol*. 64:6-8 (1989).
64. J. M. Leiper, and D. H. Lawson, Why do doctors not report adverse drug reactions? *Neth J Med* 28:546-50 (1985).

CONTRIBUTORS

Keith Beard, B.Sc., M.B., MRCP
Consultant Physician in Geriatric Medicine
Victoria Infirmary/South General
  Hospital Unit
Victoria Geriatric Unit
Mansionhouse Road
Langside Glasgow G41 3DX
SCOTLAND

Bernard Begaud, M.D.
Professor
Centre de Pharmacovigilance
Hopital Carreire-Pellegrin
Zone Nord Bat. 1A
33076 Bordeaux Cedex
FRANCE

Jeffrey L. Carson, M.D.
Associate Professor & Chief,
  Division of General Internal Medicine
UMDNJ (Univ. of Med. & Dentistry of NJ)
Room 407 - Robert Wood Johnson
  Medical School
Professional Center
97 Paterson Street
New Brunswick, NJ   08903

Terri H. Creagh, M.S., M.S.P.H.
AIDS Research Consortium of Atlanta
131 Ponce De Leon Avenue
Suite 220
Altanta, GA   30308

Henry Glick, M.A.
Research Specialist
Health Services Research
University of Pennsylvania
Section of General Internal Medicine
3615 Chestnut Street
Philadelphia, PA   19104-2676

Thomas P. Gross, M.D., M.P.H.
Section Chief, Epidemiology
Food and Drug Administration   HFD-733
Room 15-42
5600 Fisher Lane
Rockville, MD   20857

Gordon H. Guyatt, M.D.
Associate Professor of
Epidemiology and Biostatistics
McMaster University
1200 Main Street West
Room 2C12
Hamilton, Ontario, L8N 3Z5
CANADA

Judith K. Jones, M.D., Ph.D.
President
The Degge Group, Ltd.
Drug Safety Research & Information
1616 North Fort Myer Drive
Suite 1430
Arlington, VA   22209

Raynard Kington, M.D.
University of California-Los Angeles
  School of Medicine
A-671 Factor Bldg.
10833 LeConte Avenue
Los Angeles, CA   90024

R. H. B. Meyboom, M.D.
Centre for Monitoring of Adverse Reactions
  to Drugs
P.O. Box 5406,
2280 HK Rijswijk,
THE NETHERLANDS

Paul D. Stolley, M.D., M.P.H.
Professor & Chairman, Dept. of
  Epidemiology & Preventive Medicine
University of Maryland School of Medicine
655 West Baltimore Street
Baltimore, MD 21201

Brian L. Strom, M.D., M.P.H.
Associate Professor of Medicine
  and Pharmacology
Director, Clinical Epidemiology Unit
University of Pennsylvania
  School of Medicine
420 Service Drive
Room 315R - Nursing Education Bldg.
Philadelphia, PA 19104-6095

Giampaolo Velo, M.D.
Professor of Pharmacology
Director of the Institute of Pharmacology
University of Verona
Policlinico Borgo Roma
37134 Verona
ITALY

Bengt-Erik Wiholm, M.D., Ph.D.
Section of Pharmacoepidemiology
Medical Products Agency
Box 26 S-751 03 Uppsala
SWEDEN

INDEX

Accuracy, 135
Acetazolamide, 15
Acquired Immunodeficiency Syndrome,
        143-157
Adenocarcinoma of the vagina, 46, 49
Aggregate analyses, 2
Agranulocytosis, 3, 11, 16
AIDS, 143-157
Algorithm, 105, 106, 108
Ambispective cohort study, 53
Aplastic anemia, 15
Asthma, 43
Attributable risk reduction, 61
Automated databases, 54, 65-71
AZT, 143

Background equivalence, 5
Bayesian approach to evaluating a
            suspected adverse event,
            106, 108
Benoxaprofen, 22, 74
Bias, 50
Biliary duct carcinoma, 45
Bladder cancer, 45
Blinding, 60
Blood dyscrasias, 3, 11, 13, 15, 16
Boston Collaborative Drug Surveillance
        Program, 74, 84, 89, 92

Case-control studies, 49-51
Causal uncertainty, 2
Causality assessments, 10, 11, 103-113
Children, 29
Cimetidine, 2
Clinical judgment, 105
Cohort studies, 53-58
Comprehensive Hospital Drug
        Monitoring - Berne, 95
Confounding by the indication, 2, 50, 54
Confounding variable, 49
Controls for case-control studies, 49
Cost containment, 100
Cost identification analyses, 116
Cost-benefit analysis, 118
Cost-effectiveness analysis, 117

Costs, 118
Criteria for a causal association, 104
Cyclamates, 45
Cyclobenzaprine, 2

Deep vein thrombosis, 13, 14, 22, 44
DES, see Diethylstilbestrol
Descriptive studies, 93
Diethylstilbestrol, 22, 46, 49
Direct costs, 118
Discount rate, 121
Double blinding, 60
Double-masking, 60
Drug use evaluation program, 99, 100
Drug utilization studies, 92

Efficacy, 115
Efficiency, 115
Elderly, 29
Endometrial cancer, 47
Erythema multiforme, 14
Exogenous estrogens, 47

FDA, 1-7
Fixed costs, 119
France, 39-42

Generic instruments, 137
Glibenclamide, 14
Global clinical judgment, 104
Global introspection, 105
Group Health Cooperative of Puget
        Sound, 68
Guillain-Barré syndrome, 15

Halcion, 159-167
Health Maintenance Organization, 66
Health profiles, 137
Health status, 135
HELP system, 88
Hospital of the University of
        Pennsylvania, 99
Hospital surveillance, 83
Hospital-based adverse drug reaction
        monitoring, 99

Hospital-based intensive cohort studies, 91-98
Human capital approach, 120
Hydralazine, 14
Hypothesis generating studies, 75, 76, 94
Hypothesis strengthening studies, 76, 79
Hypothesis testing studies, 76, 79, 93

IHS, 85
IMS America, 2, 84
Independence, 5
Indirect costs, 120
Intention-to-treat analysis, 60

JCAHO, 99
Joint Commission on Accreditation of Health Care Organizations, 99

Kaiser Permanente, 68, 75

Lactic acidosis, 14
Latter Day Saints Hospital, 88
Lupoid reactions, 14

Marginal costs, 119
Medicaid, 68
MediMetrik, 85
Meta-analysis, 62
Methyldopa, 45

N of 1 randomized trials, 125-134
NARD, 24
Nebulizers, 43
Netherlands, 21-37
Netherlands Centre for Monitoring of Adverse Drug Reactions, 24
Nonsteroidal anti-inflammatory drugs, 2, 11
Number needed to treat, 61

Opportunity cost, 116
Oral contraceptives, 14, 22, 44

Pharmacoeconomics, 115
Pharmacosurveillance, 39
Pharmacovigilance, 39, 109
Phenformin, 14
Phocomelia, 45
Point of view, 120
Population at risk, 2
Prazosin, 2
Prescription Event Monitoring, 75
Prospective cohort study, 53
Pulmonary embolism, 44

Quality of life, 135-142
Quality of Well-Being Scale, 138
Quality-adjusted year of life, 117

Random allocation, 59
Randomized trials, 59-63
Relative risk reduction, 61
Reporting biases, 2
Representativeness, 5
Responsiveness, 137
Retrospective cohort study, 53
Reye's syndrome, 50

Saccharin, 45
Safety, 115
Salicylate, 50
Sample size requirements for case-control studies, 50
Saskatchewan Health, 68
Scientific overviews, 62
Screening, 73, 75
Sensitivity analysis, 121
Serious adverse drug reactions, 1, 10
Specific instruments, 139
Spontaneous reporting of adverse drug reactions, 1, 9, 21, 39, 74
Standard gamble, 138
Stevens-Johnson syndrome, 13
Subacute myelo-optic neuropathy (SMON), 44
Sulfasalazine, 16
Suprofen, 22, 74
Sweden, 9-20

Targeted reporting, 30
Thalidomide, 22, 45
Thromboembolic disease, 13, 14, 22, 44
Ticrynafen, 74
Time trade off, 138
Triazolam, 159-167

Underreporting, 2
Utility measurement, 138

Validity, 135
Variable costs, 119
Vital statistics, 43

Walsh Hospital Drug and Diagnostic Index, 85
Willingness-to-pay, 120

Zidovudine, 143
Zomepirac, 74